# The Origin and Development of Genetic Therapies

*From Magic and Superstition to Molecular Genetics and the Human Genome*

THEODORE FRIEDMANN
*Professor of Pediatrics, Emeritus, UCSD School of Medicine*

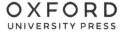

# OXFORD
UNIVERSITY PRESS

Oxford University Press is a department of the University of Oxford.
It furthers the University's objective of excellence in research, scholarship,
and education by publishing worldwide. Oxford is a registered trade mark of
Oxford University Press in the UK and certain other countries.

Published in the United States of America by Oxford University Press
198 Madison Avenue, New York, NY 10016, United States of America.

© Theodore Friedmann 2025

All rights reserved. No part of this publication may be reproduced, stored in a retrieval system, transmitted, used for text and data mining, or used for training artificial intelligence, in any form or by any means, without the prior permission in writing of Oxford University Press, or as expressly permitted by law, by license or under terms agreed with the appropriate reprographics rights organization. Inquiries concerning reproduction outside the scope of the above should be sent to the Rights Department, Oxford University Press, at the address above.

You must not circulate this work in any other form
and you must impose this same condition on any acquirer.

Library of Congress Cataloging-in-Publication Data
Names: Friedmann, Theodore, 1935- author.
Title: The origin and development of genetic therapies : from magic and
superstition to molecular genetics and the human genome / Theodore Friedmann.
Description: New York, NY : Oxford University Press, [2025] | Includes index.
Identifiers: LCCN 2025002395 (print) | LCCN 2025002396 (ebook) |
ISBN 9780197689974 (paperback) | ISBN 9780197689981 (updf) |
ISBN 9780197689998 (epub) | ISBN 9780197690000 (online)
Subjects: MESH: Genetic Therapy—history
Classification: LCC RB155 (print) | LCC RB155 (ebook) | NLM QU 11.1 |
DDC 616/.042—dc23/eng/20250408
LC record available at https://lccn.loc.gov/2025002395
LC ebook record available at https://lccn.loc.gov/2025002396

This material is not intended to be, and should not be considered, a substitute for medical or other professional advice. Treatment for the conditions described in this material is highly dependent on the individual circumstances. And, while this material is designed to offer accurate information with respect to the subject matter covered and to be current as of the time it was written, research and knowledge about medical and health issues is constantly evolving and dose schedules for medications are being revised continually, with new side effects recognized and accounted for regularly. Readers must therefore always check the product information and clinical procedures with the most up-to-date published product information and data sheets provided by the manufacturers and the most recent codes of conduct and safety regulation. The publisher and the authors make no representations or warranties to readers, express or implied, as to the accuracy or completeness of this material. Without limiting the foregoing, the publisher and the authors make no representations or warranties as to the accuracy or efficacy of the drug dosages mentioned in the material. The authors and the publisher do not accept, and expressly disclaim, any responsibility for any liability, loss or risk that may be claimed or incurred as a consequence of the use and/ or application of any of the contents of this material.

DOI: 10.1093/med/9780197689974.001.0001

Printed by Integrated Books International, United States of America

The manufacturer's authorized representative in the EU for product safety is
Oxford University Press España S.A., Parque Empresarial San Fernando de Henares,
Avenida de Castilla, 2 – 28830 Madrid (www.oup.es/en).

# Acknowledgement

"I dedicate this book to Ingrid, my love and my inspiration".

I also thank my colleagues who reviewed early drafts of the book and who made many helpful suggestions on what I should include and how to present it—Thomas Gelehrter, Erling Norrby, Carl Johan Sundberg, Paul Friedmann, Marc Schuckit.

I am especially grateful to my mentors and friends who have pointed me as best they could in the direction of rigorous science—Fred Sanger, Christian Anfinsen, J. Edwin Seegmiller, Renato Dulbecco and Arne Ljungqvist.

# Contents

Introduction: emergence of scientific therapies—the birth of a new kind of therapy ... 1

1. Early Western concepts of disease and therapy ... 3
2. From Galen to the Renaissance—anatomy and the cell and germ theories ... 9
3. Darwin, Mendel and Galton—the discovery, disappearance and rediscovery of the laws of inheritance ... 21
4. The rediscovery of Mendel, Garrod and human biochemical genetics ... 31
5. Mutations are inherited by Mendel's laws and can cause disease. What are chromosomes? What elements in chromosomes cause disease?—The Sutton-Boveri chromosome theory ... 37
6. DNA is the repository and transmitter of genetic information ... 41
7. From inborn errors to molecular disease ... 53
8. First faltering steps toward gene therapy—viruses as gene transfer vectors ... 61
9. Birth of molecular biology and recombinant DNA—the remarkable 1960s–1970s ... 67
10. Potential misstep becomes reality—the emergence of federal oversight and regulation ... 85
11. Oversight and regulation of recombinant DNA research—the Asilomar conferences ... 91
12. Chemical nonviral vectors ... 99
13. Genetics—from a descriptive to a manipulative science ... 105
14. Early clinical gene therapy trials ... 119

| | |
|---|---|
| 15. From academia to the bedside—the design of clinical trials | 127 |
| 16. The Human Genome Project—a complement, but not the origin, of gene therapy | 131 |
| 17. A third serious setback | 135 |
| 18. Finally—breakthrough success? | 141 |
| 19. Gene editing—a foundational new era for genetic therapies | 155 |
| 20. RNA-based therapies and programmable RNA editing | 171 |
| 21. The role of biotech and pharma in the development of gene therapy | 175 |
| 22. Current dilemma and future directions | 181 |
| 23. Summary: genetic therapies—a new field of medicine | 189 |
| *Index* | 193 |

# Introduction: emergence of scientific therapies—the birth of a new kind of therapy

The 20th century witnessed the birth of an entirely new field of medicine that was unlike all previous concepts of medicine and therapeutics (i.e., gene therapy). It became possible for the first time to use the vast body of scientific understanding of living systems accumulated over the millennia, especially the 19th and 20th centuries, not only to understand the underlying causes and nature of human disease but also to make fundamental changes in human biology that could mitigate the forces that cause disease.

At the heart of that revolutionary conceptual change were the remarkable birth and growth of genetics and its shift from a purely descriptive to a powerfully manipulative science that promises and threatens to redesign human biology and human evolution. The pace of that shift has been remarkably fast, making it difficult to try to predict the many ways, for good and for ill, in which the technology will move. But certainly, the improved management of human disease will be a major beneficiary of this scientific explosion.

To appreciate the historical forces underlying this change and to underscore how epochal the birth and development of modern genetic medicine has been, I wish in this book to chronicle, at least briefly, the origins of medical therapeutics from ancient times until present day. Given the speed with which genetics is changing human biology and human medicine, the purpose of this account is not to review all of the current ongoing advances but rather to try to review where and how the field of genetic medicine arose and how it is changing what we understand of disease and how our concepts of the causes and treatments of human disease have and continue to change now with ever increasing and startling speed. In the blink of an eye, we have moved from discovering that there is a genetic basis for much of human disease to being able to control some genetic disease by adding normal genetic information to diseased cells and tissues or to change or "edit" the resident and disease-causing genetic information. Those approaches have until very recently not been designed to truly correct the underlying genetic defect—rather they merely circumvent the pathogenic mechanisms. Until now! With the advent of genetic editing, there is now the completely new opportunity to definitively "fix what is broken"—to re-design aberrant gene or, for that matter, to redesign much of human biology and evolution.

# 1
# Early Western concepts of disease and therapy

Modern Western medical thinking and concepts of disease and treatment are largely derived from the thinking of the ancient Greeks more than three millennia ago. A prevailing concept of health and illness at that time was that all matter in Nature consisted of four basic elements—earth, water, air, and fire—and that the harmony of the world required that those elements needed to be in balance. By analogy, human health and well-being required not only that the elements of the world be balanced but also that four basic liquids or "humors" of life—blood, phlegm, yellow bile, and black bile—be in harmony. Keeping these four humors in balance was the key to good health and happiness and bringing them back into harmony was the goal of treatment of disease. Just how that was to be achieved was unclear but often was based on magic, superstition, or sacrificial offerings to angered gods. It was believed that disease resulted from the vengeance of aggrieved gods who caused disharmony of the life humors and who could be assuaged through spiritual, religious and superstitious approaches.

As early as the 6th and 7th centuries BC, medical cults and their teachings began to emerge. Probably the first of these was the school of the philosopher Alcmaeon at Cnidus (ca. 500 BC). The prevailing concepts of disease and its treatment at that time included some teachings from the more advanced traditions of Egyptian medicine and included the idea of disease stemming from disharmony between the opposing body powers (wet/dry, hot/cold, sweet/sour, etc.) and retribution of displeased gods. But more worldly and rational schools of medical thought emerged in Greece from 600 to 500 BC that taught that superstitious and magical approaches to illness should be countered by understanding the material basis of illness and by emphasizing the science underlying the harmony of the human body with the external world, stressing the connection between a healthy body and the healthy mind. The major schools of ancient Greek medicine included the cult surrounding the demigod Asklepios (mid-300 BC) (identified as Aesculapius in later Roman iterations), the Greco-Roman philosopher-healer Hippocrates of Kos (460–370 BC) and Claudius Galenus or Galen of Pergamon (129–216 AD), a major follower of Hippocrates later to become physician to Roman emperors.

**AESCULAPIUS** (Figure 1.1). The partial human–partial demigod Aesculapius was the son of Apollo, and his cult and school of healing emerged

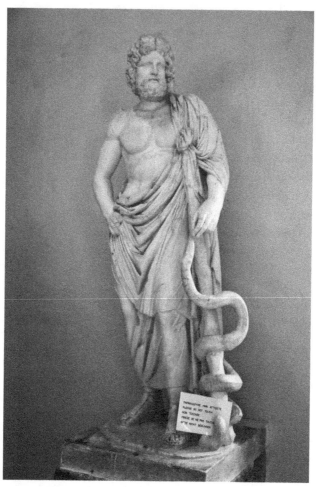

**Figure 1.1.** Aesculapius
Aesculapius. Greek god of Medicine, son of Apollo. Aesculapius was killed by Zeus to prevent him from making men immortal. Reproduced from Michael F. Mehnert, CC BY-SA 3.0 <https://creativecommons.org/licenses/by-sa/3.0>, via Wikimedia Commons.

during the period from about 300 BC. The Aesculapian healing cult became popular and attracted many to his healing centers seeking to treat their illnesses and even to bring the dead back to life, using ritual purifications, incantations and sacrificial offerings to repel evil spirits and appease the angered gods. Healing therefore was primarily an exercise in countering supernatural forces and appeasing angered gods and not so much on rational observation. Aesculapius himself came to be represented by a walking rod and by a snake, wound around the rod, that represented fertility and rebirth because of its ability to shed its skin and re-emerge in renewed form, and through the likely use of snakes in sacrificial offerings.

**HIPPOCRATES** (ca. 460–370 BC) (Figure 1.2). Hippocrates from the Greek island of Kos lived from about 460 BC to 370 BC. At the time when illness was usually attributed to superstition and retribution of wrathful gods,

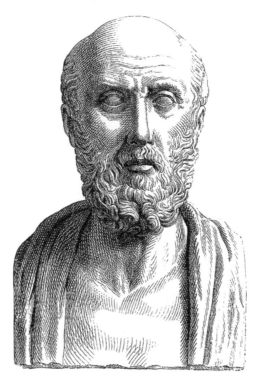

**Figure 1.2.** Hippocrates
Hippocrates. (460–370 BC). Greek physician and philosopher—considered by many to be the "Father of Medicine." Reproduced from 1881 *Young Persons' Cyclopedia of Persons and Places*, Engraving.

Hippocrates taught that the human being comprised a soul and a body and that good health required the two to be in harmony. He further taught that human illness was not the result of godly retribution or demons but rather had a natural cause and that in order to treat illness, it would be necessary to understand that connection with nature. He further taught that those natural causes could be identified by observation and study of Nature and an understanding of how disturbances of Nature bring the body humors into disarray, thereby causing disease. That required understanding of the unique life circumstances and history of each person—truly the beginnings of "evidence-based" medicine. Because disease results from disturbed forces of nature, natural cures might also be used to prevent and treat disease. This more rational concept of disease and treatment included exercise and a healthy diet to promote a healthy mind in a healthy body. Treatments were holistic and even included music and drama for treatment. For instance, alternating flute and harp sounds were thought to be beneficial in the treatment of gout.

Through this emphasis on a more rational approach to understanding disease and the beginnings of natural approaches to treatment, Hippocrates has become identified as the "father of medicine." His teachings were compiled and codified into the Hippocratic Corpus assembled in Alexandria, Egypt, during the third century BC. In modern times, he has come to be remembered for his ethical teachings to healers in what is known as the "Hippocratic Oath." As all modern medical practitioners learn, among his writings appears this famous admonition to healers taken from Hippocrates' "Epidemics I":

*Read the past, diagnose the present, foretell the future; practice these acts. As to diseases, make a habit of two things—to help, or at least to do no harm."*

**GALEN** (129–216 AD) (Figure 1.3). Galen, unlike Aesculapius and Hippocrates, was not only a believer in the Hippocratic concepts of humoral imbalance as a cause of human illness but also sought more actively to find new drugs and medicines that could restore a more healthful balance to the body humors. Galen and his followers carried further the Hippocratic emphasis on observation of Nature and stressed the importance of animal experimentation and dissection. Just as Hippocrates is considered a father of rational observation of Nature, Galen can be thought of as the originator of the concept of experimental medicine, as part of his emphasis on the animal

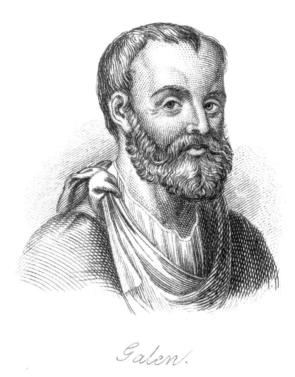

**Figure 1.3.** Galen
Galen (Claudius Galenus) (129–216). Greco-Roman physician, philosopher and researcher, pioneer of the value of animal dissection and anatomy. Reproduced with permission from *Portraits of Doctors and Scientists in the Wellcome Institute of the History of Medicine. A Catalogue*, by Renate Burgess, London, Wellcome Institute of the History of Medicine, 1973, pp. xxiv, 459. Copyright © Cambridge University Press, 1974.

dissection and experimentation for understanding disease. That emphasis led him to discover that urine was produced in the kidney and to prove the blood-carrying role of arteries and veins, although the concept of blood circulation eluded him and awaited the work of William Harvey in the 17th century. In this role as an experimentalist and anatomist, he studied the function of the pulse and the use of the pulse as an indicator of the state of a person's health. He also invented a novel formulation for the herbal jam Theriac, the wonder drug of the time, that was used as an antidote for snake bites and a cure-all for other ailments. Theriac in its many variations and formulations was used even as late as the 19th century.

While these early fathers of medicine developed these disparate approaches to the treatment of disease, there is little reference to familial occurrences of disease and what, if anything, that might reveal of the causes of illness or suggest for treatment. There was therefore little or no understanding of heritable disease and what exactly it was that was common to people in families suffering from similar illnesses that might suggest treatments. Hippocrates himself taught that physical traits were inherited through sperm, but a direct connection with disease was not made in his teachings or those of Aesculapius or Galen.

# 2
# From Galen to the Renaissance—anatomy and the cell and germ theories

During the long dark ages that enveloped the world after Galen, advances in understanding the cause and treatment of human disease were slow and minimal, especially from the vantage point of Western medicine. But during the Middle Ages from the 7th to 14th centuries, a major body of scientific and medical thinking was developing in the Muslim world, even superseding the Greco-Roman teachings, particularly in human anatomy (1) more so than in the causes and treatment of human disease. Islamic scholars including Al-Razi/Razes (865–925 AD), Ali Ibn Abbas/Haly Abbas (? 930–994 AD), Al-Baghdadi (1162–1231 AD) and others made major advances in anatomy and corrected many of the inaccuracies and mistakes in the Galenic anatomical teachings that resulted from Galen's anatomical concepts based entirely on dissections of monkeys and other animals rather than of humans. However, in contrast to anatomy, there was much less innovation and progress in that Islamic medicine toward an understanding of the causes and treatment of human disease.

With the emergence in Europe of the Renaissance in the 15th and 16th centuries, the arts, science and medical thinking began to flourish in Europe, overtaking the Islamic teachings. Through the work of the Polish astronomer Nicolaus Copernicus (1473–1543) and the Italian Galileo Galilei (1564–1642), the modern science of astronomy was born that disproved the Ptolemaic teaching that the Earth was the center of the universe and that showed that it was the Sun rather than the Earth that was the center of our world. Medical treatments moved away from the herbal cures developed by the Islamic physicians and toward therapies such as the disease-specific therapy developed by the German physician Paracelsus (Philippus Aureolus Theophrastus Bombast von Hohenheim) (1493–1541), known as Paracelsus for recommending drinking mercury to cure syphilis. These new ideas of treatment became available in church-based hospitals for the vast number of the sick suffering from epidemics and infectious diseases.

The explosion of studies of human disease, anatomy and physiology during the Renaissance in Europe reflected the extensive human dissections carried out by the great painters and sculptors of the Renaissance Leonardo da Vinci and Michelangelo Buonarroti and the later anatomists Andreas Vesalius and William Harvey.

As in almost everything that he touched, Leonardo Da Vinci revolutionized the understanding of human anatomy through his dissections and his art (Figure 2.1).

Similarly, the artist Michelangelo Buonarroti (1475–1564) understood human anatomy far better than previous anatomists but confined himself almost exclusively to the human musculoskeletal system and not at all to human disease (see Figure 2.2).

The most important early Western experimental anatomists were the 16th-century Dutch Andreas Vesalius (1514–1564) (see Figure 2.3), who described his revolutionary studies in *De Humanis Corporis Fabrica Libri Septem* in 1543, and the late 16th- and early 17th-century English anatomist William Harvey, who discovered and reported in 1628 that the function of the heart is to pump blood through the body and that it was the function of the veins to return blood to the heart (see Figure 2.4). Those discoveries disproved one and a half millennia of Galenic teaching. As important as these studies were to an understanding of the structural aspects of some human diseases, they had little or no relevance to questions of the origins and treatments of most human diseases.

Additional significant advances toward a truly scientific understanding of the underlying causes of disease during the Renaissance began to emerge with the invention by the Dutch draper Antonie van Leeuwenhoek (1632–1723) (Figure 2.5) of the microscope and his resulting discovery of individual cells as the structural basis of life (see Figure 2.6). He was the first to describe red blood cells, spermatozoa, muscle fibers, bacteria (that he called "animalcules") and to describe the flow of blood through capillaries, all of which he documented in many letters to the Royal Society of Science in England.

At approximately the same time, Robert Hooke (1635–1703), the English philosopher, inventor, physicist, architect and microscopist, and assistant to Robert Boyle who had discovered the pressure–volume relationship of gases (Boyle's Law), invented and used a more advanced compound microscope version of the more primitive Leeuwenhoek instrument to discover the boxlike structures in cork and other plants that he called "cells," thereby

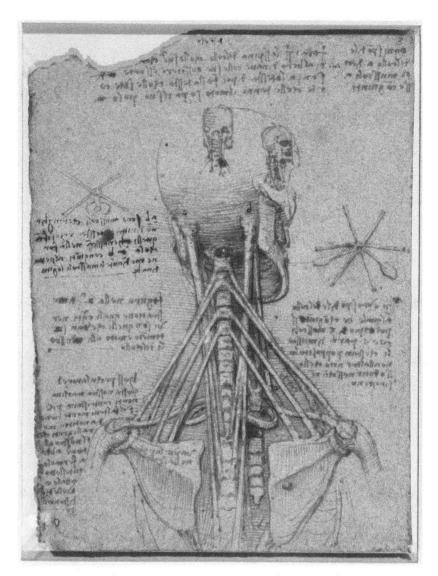

**Figure 2.1.** Neck dissection by Leonardo da Vinci (1452–1519). Renaissance polymath–inventor, artist. Reproduced with permission from Royal Collection Trust, Copyright © His Majesty King Charles III 2024.

opening the door and giving name to a theory that living things were composed of these small basic subunits—cells (see Figure 2.7). He reported his many microscopic life observations of fungi, protozoa and plants in his 1665 book *Micrographia* and in many letters to the English Royal Society.

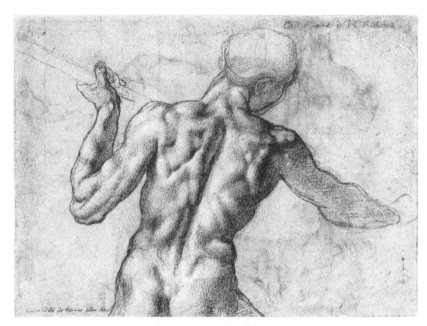

**Figure 2.2.** Michelangelo Buonarroti (1475–1564). Italian Renaissance painter, sculptor and architect. Male Back with a Flag, Michelangelo.

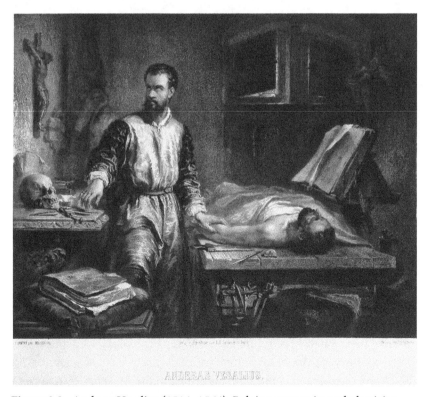

**Figure 2.3.** Andreas Vesalius (1514–1564). Belgian anatomist and physician, founder of human anatomy. Reproduced from lithograph by E. Milster after E.J.C. Hamman, 1849. Wellcome Collection.

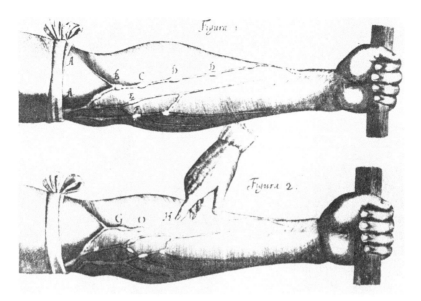

**Figure 2.4.** William Harvey (1578–1657). English physician and physiologist, discoverer of blood circulation, demonstrating venous return of blood. Reproduced from Sigerist, Henry E. (1965) Große Ärzte, München, Deutschland: J.F. Lehmans Verlag (5. Auflage) (1. Auflage 1958) plate 26 p 120.

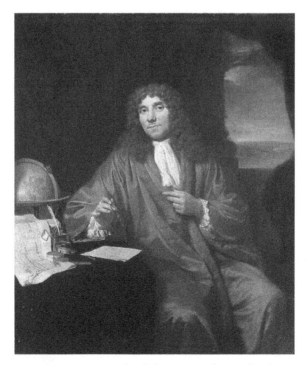

**Figure 2.5.** Antonie van Leeuwenhoek (1632–1723). Dutch microscopist and microbiologist, discoverer of microorganisms ("animalcules"). Reproduced from Physicist at Delft, Jan Verkolje (I), 1680–1686, oil on canvas, h 56 cm × w 47.5 cm. Source: http://hdl.handle.net/10934/RM0001.COLLECT.7080

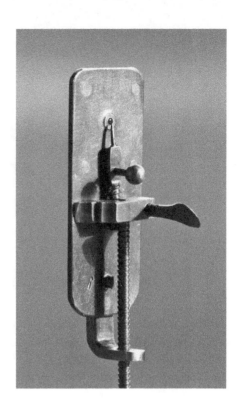

**Figure 2.6.** Early model microscope of Antonie van Leeuwenhoek. Photograph by Jeroen Rouwkema. Reproduced under the CC BY-NC-ND 2.0 DEED license: https://creativecommons.org/licenses/by-nc-nd/2.0/

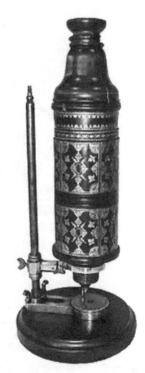

**Figure 2.7.** Microscope of Robert Hooke (1635–1703). English physicist, astronomer, geologist, architect. Hooke used a compound microscope to discover the compartment-like structure of cork that he likened to "cells" of a honeycomb, laying the foundation for cell theory of living organisms.

He is, together with Leeuwenhoek, legitimately recognized as a father of microbiology.

The discovery that living matter, both animal and plant, consisted of basic elemental units of "cells" was established and fully accepted from the work of a series of mostly German/Polish scientists in the mid-late 19th century, principal among whom were Matthias Schleiden (1804–1881), Theodor Schwann (1810–1882) and Rudolf Virchow (1821–1902). Especially important was the work of Schleiden and Schwann, who established that all forms of life, animal or plant, consisted of elemental subunits of cells. But it is fair to say that, although the concepts and proofs of cellular pathology were established by this school of scientists, it was the discoveries of Virchow that were especially important and have earned him the title of "father of cellular pathology." Virchow taught that all cells arise from previously existing cells and that disease did not reflect abnormal function of an entire organism but rather resulted from the abnormal function of specific cells in the body. That concept brought him into conflict with the concept emerging from the work of biologists such as Louis Pasteur who believed that at least some human disease is caused by infection with outside agents—microorganisms. Of course, both concepts are now known to be correct.

However important the observations on the cell basis of life, they did little if anything to illuminate the function of these structures nor their possible relationship to disease. That was to come two centuries later with the maturation of the world of microbiology and the discovery of microbes and their role in human illness. Among the major pioneers in this development were the English physician Edward Jenner, French scientist Louis Pasteur, the German microbiologist Robert Koch, the English surgeon Joseph Lister and the Austro-Hungarian Ignaz Semmelweiss.

One of the earliest demonstrations of the role of microscopic life in human disease involved keen clinical observation and astute intuition and did not rely at all on the demonstration of a microscopic organism. Edward Jenner (1749–1823) was an English physician who noticed that milkmaids who had been exposed to cows with the pustules of a smallpox-like disease of cows (variolae vaccinae) never seemed to develop full-blown smallpox (see Figure 2.8).

He postulated that material in the cow pustules might protect against smallpox. He did not conjecture on exactly what was the nature of the agent in the pustule that was responsible for causing the infection, but he intuited

16  ORIGIN AND DEVELOPMENT OF GENETIC THERAPIES

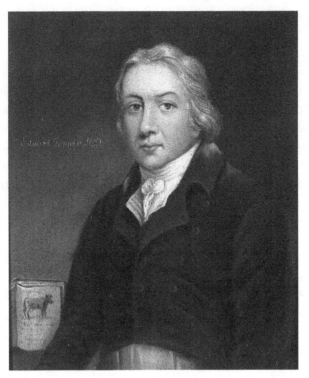

**Figure 2.8.** Edward Jenner (1749–1823), English physician and developer of the first designed "vaccine." He called his procedure "vaccination" in honor of the cow source of the inoculating material ("vaca" in Latin). Reproduced from Edward Jenner, Oil painting, Wellcome Collection 47332i.

that since the disease was infectious and the pustule was the most obvious manifestation of the disease, the responsible agent could reside there. In a stroke of genius, he inferred that the material in pustules not only caused disease but conceivably could be used to protect against infection by inoculation into healthy people. Indeed, the concept of inoculation with disease material was not entirely new at the time and was in some use in Africa and Asia. He obviously did not have the help of microscopic visualization of the pathogen—he would not have seen anything since the smallpox pathogen is a submicroscopic virus. Nevertheless, he acted on his intuition and inoculated the young son of his gardener and additional subjects with material from cowpox pustules. Remarkably, those inoculated people did not contract smallpox. What Jenner proved in this and subsequent experiments was that after subsequent challenge with cowpox material, the recipients did not develop any disease symptoms and became immune to smallpox. In recognition of the discovery, in 1796 Jenner called the process of protecting humans from this infectious agent "vaccination" in honor of the source of the therapeutic material—Latin "vacca" for cow.

Louis Pasteur (see Figure 2.9) was a French chemist commonly considered a father of microbiology whose work put an end to the two-millennia-old idea espoused by Aristotle that life arises spontaneously from nonliving matter (spontaneous generation). He provided vital evidence supporting the germ theory of human disease and developed the process of heat treatment of milk (pasteurization) to inactivate pathogenic microbes in the milk.

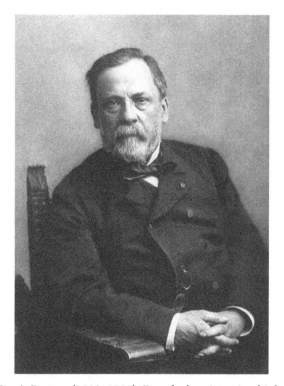

Figure 2.9. Louis Pasteur (1822–1895), French chemist, microbiologist. Pasteur popularized the germ theory of disease and the prophylactic use of vaccines to prevent disease. Reproduced from photogravure by Photographische Gesellschaft, Berlin (photographic company), published by Photographische Gesellschaft, Berlin (photographic company). Collection: Scientific Identity. Smithsonian Libraries. SIL-SIL14-p002-04.

Pasteur's contemporary counterpart and cofounder of medical microbiology was the German physician Robert Koch, the first scientist to prove that a microbe was the immediate cause of a human infectious disease through his discovery of the agent and spore cycle of the anthrax bacterium (see Figure 2.10). He also discovered the agent responsible for tuberculosis, and through his discovery of asymptomatic carriers of cholera and typhus, he developed the famous "Koch postulates" for the development of human clinical infectious disease—human infections disease—a candidate pathogen must be present in all cases of a disease, it must be isolatable and grown in the laboratory, it must recapitulate the naturally occurring disease when inoculated into healthy animals and it must then be re-isolated in a form identical to the originally isolated agent.

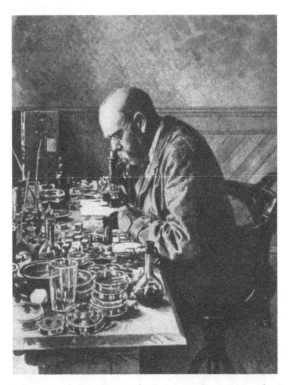

**Figure 2.10.** Robert Koch (1843–1910). German physician and microbiologist, a founder of modern microbiology and discoverer of infectious agents responsible for tuberculosis, cholera and anthrax. Reproduced from KRUIF, Paul de. Mikrobenjäger. Orell Füssli, Zürich, 1927.

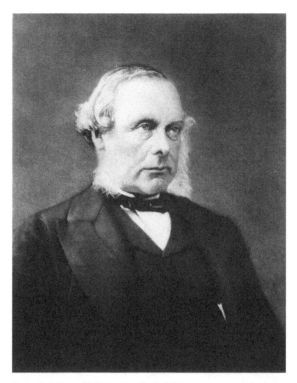

**Figure 2.11.** Joseph Lister (1827–1912). British surgeon and pioneer of antiseptic techniques for surgery. Reproduced from Wellcome Collection. Reference: 14444i.

These discoveries led quickly to the application of the microbial basis for human illness to the world of surgery, where wound infections were a constant and dangerous problem. The English surgeon Joseph Lister (see Figure 2.11) was inspired by Louis Pasteur's discoveries and developed a method for disinfecting the surgical instruments and dressings with a spray of phenol, thereby dramatically reducing the incidence of wound infection and establishing himself as the father of modern aseptic surgery.

Even simpler but equally elegant was the concept developed by the Austro-Hungarian physician Ignaz Semmelweiss (1818–1865) (see Figure 2.12) that the all-too-common obstetrical infections following childbirth (puerperal fever) were caused by microbial infection but could be prevented by the simple act of careful handwashing with chlorinated water. His ideas were slow to gain acceptance by his colleagues and he was roundly rejected for multiple academic hospital positions. Ironically, Semmelweiss finally

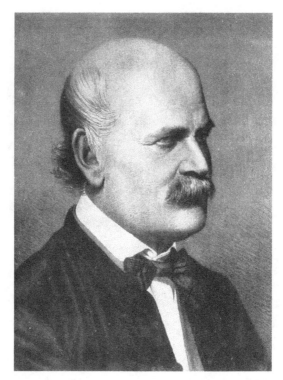

**Figure 2.12.** Ignaz Semmelweiss (1818–1865). Hungarian-Viennese physician and pioneer in antiseptic care during childbirth, emphasizing simple handwashing to prevent puerperal postpartum infection. Copper plate engraving by Jenő Doby (1860).

had what seemed to be an emotional breakdown and was involuntarily institutionalized, still more-or-less under-appreciated and embittered by his colleagues' rejection of his revolutionary work simply because it contradicted their established and entrenched teachings. He died shortly afterward of sepsis caused by an infected hand wound—ironically, the same illness which he worked so hard to prevent in the obstetric service in Vienna.

### Reference

1. Alghamdi MA, Ziermann JM, Diogo R. An untold story: The important contributions of Muslim scholars for the understanding of human anatomy. American Association for Anatomy. Nov. 2016, https://doi.org/10.1002/ar.23523

# 3
# Darwin, Mendel and Galton—the discovery, disappearance and rediscovery of the laws of inheritance

The discovery of genetics in 19th-century England did not occur in an intellectual or scientific vacuum but instead arose in the context of the scientific turmoil of earth-shaking development of the concept of natural selection driven through biological evolution as expounded by Charles Darwin (1809–1882) (see Figure 3.1) in his work, *On the Origin of Species*, published in 1859.

Darwin demonstrated that biological systems and organisms arise from predecessor systems and change and evolve as a result of selection of inherited variants that confer advantage to compete, survive and therefore to reproduce. Of course, he had no knowledge of the genetic mechanisms that drive biological variation, how genetic variants arise, how some are selected for, others discarded and how genetic traits are transmitted from one generation to the next. But his work firmly established the concepts of developmental and evolutionary genetics and laid the groundwork for all the genetic discoveries of genetic inheritance that flowed quickly on the heels of his work.

Darwin's cousin Francis Galton (1822–1911) (see Figure 3.2) recognized the potential relevance of Darwin's theory to human evolution and became interested in human intelligence. In 1869, Galton published *Hereditary Genius*, in which he postulated the unusual concept that mental traits, like physical human traits, are inherited, leading him eventually to propose an approach to bettering human beings by a program of selected parental selection and breeding, for which in 1883 he coined the term "eugenics," from the Greek "eu" meaning good and "genics" meaning coming into being.

Galton's view of eugenics was the positive one of selective encouragement of mating of the most fit and socially "desirable," and the concept spread widely throughout Europe and the United States. But sadly, the term came to

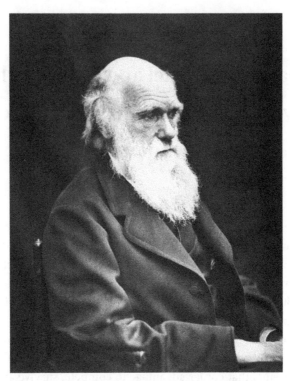

**Figure 3.1.** Charles Darwin (1809–1882). English naturalist and evolutionary biologist. Author of seminal 1859 treatise *On the Origin of Species*. Reproduced with permission from Bettmann/Bettmann Collection via Getty Images.

take on the opposite and much more sinister purpose of forcibly preventing reproduction and even extinguishing the life of humans considered "unfit to live and unfit to reproduce." This negative meaning of eugenics spread widely in the early 20th century as promulgated by Charles Davenport and Harry Laughlin, the founder and director, respectively, of the Eugenics Record Office of the Cold Spring Harbor Laboratory in New York. This darker meaning of the concept of eugenics took place in the United States during the stigmatization of increasing numbers of eastern European and Asian immigrants into the United States, and many of the negative traits thought to be more common in these immigrant populations such as poverty, prostitution, criminality and intellectual deficiencies were attributed by regressive and xenophobic critics and eugenicists to genetic causes, which they argued were undesirable in the U.S. gene pool. Bizarre as it is by modern genetic and sociological understanding, these concepts were based on the

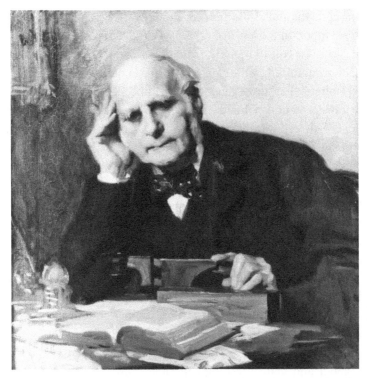

**Figure 3.2.** Francis Galton (1822–1911). Cousin of Charles Darwin, polymath and discoverer of identification potential of human fingerprints. Galton was the originator of the concept of selective breeding of humans (eugenics). Reproduced with permission from Bettmann/Bettmann Collection via Getty Images.

application of genetic concepts of the day, as incorrect and unfounded as they were. The concepts needed rationalization, accomplished at times by invention of pseudoscientific terminology. Because it was widely recognized that since many sea captains were men, the term of "thalassophilia" was even invented for the "masculine" love of the sea.

The new pseudoscientific eugenic thinking led to discriminatory sociopolitical programs such as discriminatory immigration policies and even compulsory human sterilization of "undesirables" in the United States and even in some European countries. Involuntary sterilization was even endorsed by the U.S. Supreme Court in the infamous *Buck v. Bell* decision of 1927. A young woman named Carrie Buck was institutionalized and condemned to involuntary sterilization under a new sterilization law in the state of Virginia for being epileptic and feeble minded, although she was neither of those. She was merely poor. In *Buck v. Bell* (1927), the U.S. Supreme Court ruled that Virginia's law was constitutional and that Buck should be sterilized, with the judgment pronounced by the chief justice, the famed American jurist Oliver Wendel Holmes, that "three generations of imbeciles is enough."

This transformation of the eugenics concept from being merely misguided to being overtly evil was most notoriously driven by the Nazi governments in Germany in their genocidal programs of the early-mid 20th century. Interestingly, the German sterilization programs were a legacy partly of the work of the Cold Spring Harbor laboratory and the U.S. Supreme Court *Buck v. Bell* decision, as indicated by the award by the University of Heidelberg of an honorary degree in 1936 to Harry Laughlin for his work in advancing "the science of race hygiene."

The growth of such negative eugenic policies has irretrievably tainted the history of genetics in the late 19th and early-mid 20th centuries and poisoned the well of possible modern futuristic proposed positive applications of directed human evolution, such as those implicit in some interpretations of some current manipulations of human genome editing.

At approximately the same time and quite independent of Darwin, the monk, abbot and plant breeding experimentalist Gregor Mendel (1822–1884) (see Figure 3.3) at the Augustinian St. Thomas Abbey in the provincial town of Brno in Austro-Hungary set about to study the evolution and development of the easily studied model system of pea plants. He reported the results of the studies that he carried out in the small garden outside the St. Thomas Abbey with the inheritance patterns and dominance or recessiveness of seven physical traits including pea shape, pea color, pod shape, pod color, flower color, plant size and position of flowers of pea plants to the Natural Science Society in Brno (see Figure 3.4). In 1866, the scientific society published Mendel's work in their obscure journal *Proceedings of the Brünn Society for the Study of Natural Science* under the title "Experiments on Plant Hybrids."

To say that Mendel's studies created a scientific sensation or even wide interest in the scientific community would be an exaggeration. In reality, Mendel's work and his published report were barely noticed and were greeted, if at all, with a scientific yawn. His work virtually vanished from view and failed to influence biological science for the ensuing 35 years. The laws of inheritance discovered by Gregor Mendel re-emerged at the end of the 19th century and were reported in 1900, largely through the work of a group of

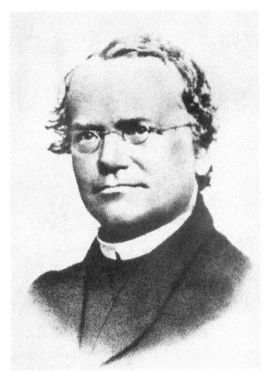

**Figure 3.3.** Gregor Mendel (1822–1884), Austrian-Czech biologist and Augustinian friar and abbot of the St. Thomas Abbey in Brno. Mendel first discovered laws of inheritance, thereby founding the science of genetics. Reproduced from National Institutes of Health.

three German, Dutch and Austrian botanists. Probably, the most important of these scientists was the Dutchman Hugo Marie de Vries (Figure 3.5), who seems to have taken inspiration from Darwin's 1868 theory of "Pangenesis." Through his plant breeding studies, de Vries proposed in his "Intracellular Pangenesis" that dominance and recessiveness, and the inheritability of trait ratios, were inherited through particles that he termed "pangenes." De Vries coined the term "mutation" to describe sudden and unexpected changes in primrose plants (De Vries, *Comptes Rendus*, March 26, 1900) as evidence for the emergence of new species by sudden mutational changes and that those acquired traits were then inherited in ways similar to those proposed by the 18th-century French zoologist Jean-Baptiste Lamarck. To underscore the importance of De Vries' attribution of mutations in the common evening primrose, its Latin name became *Oenothera lamarckia*. Interestingly,

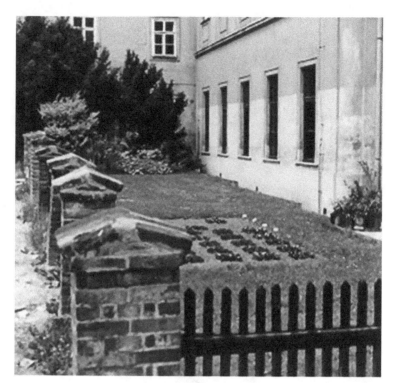

**Figure 3.4.** The garden of the St. Thomas Abbey in Brno. This is the birthplace of the science of genetics. Courtesy of Theodore Friedmann.

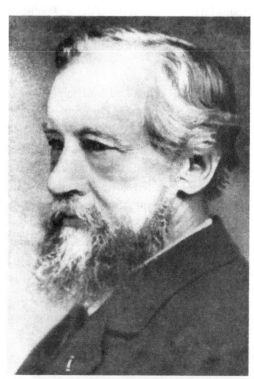

**Figure 3.5.** Hugo Marie de Vries (1848–1935). Dutch botanist and one of the discoverers of the laws of inheritance as described by Gregor Mendel. Reproduced from Hans Stubbe: *Kurze Geschichte der Genetik bis zur Wiederentdeckung Gregor Mendels* Jena, 2. Auflage 1965. Quelle dort: aus Dahlgren:BotanischeGenetik.

the interesting and even important Lamarkian concept of inheritance of acquired traits underlay the disastrously failed farming programs in the Soviet Union and did so much to destroy genetic science in that country in the 20th century. There is little or no evidence that de Vries was aware of Mendel's work, and it is likely therefore that he came to his conclusions quite independently. The De Vries term "pangenes" would later be shortened by the Danish botanist and geneticist Wilhelm Johansen to "genes" in his 1905 book *The Elements of Heredity*. Further to his generally unappreciated role as the father of much of modern genetic terminology, Johansen also first used the terms "genotype" and "phenotype" in his 1909 book *The Elements of the Exact Theory of Heredity*.

Similarly, but working independently of De Vries, the Austrian plant botanist Erich von Tschermak (1871–1962) (Figure 3.6) was studying features of pea breeding, and in 1900 he reported that his results were similar to, and could be explained by, the laws of inheritance that had been described by Gregor Mendel (*Ztschr. f. d. landw. Versuchswesen in Oesterr*). Interestingly,

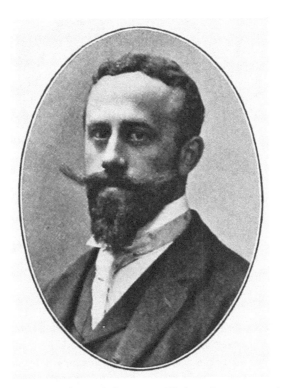

**Figure 3.6.** Erich von Tschermak (1871–1962). Austrian agronomist who rediscovered and who in 1900 published a description of Mendel's laws of genetic inheritance. Reproduced from *Acta horti bergiani* bd. III, no.3 (1905).

it seems that Tschermak's maternal grandfather, the famous botanist Eduard Fenzl, was one of Gregor Mendel's early teachers.

The third simultaneous rediscoverer of Mendel's studies was the German botanist Karl Franz Joseph Correns (1864–1933) (see Figure 3.7), who was a student of the botanist Karl Nägeli at the University of Tübingen in Germany and who had communicated with Mendel to some extent about Mendel's studies with peas, thereby possibly making Correns aware of Mendel's work. In 1900, Correns published his paper, "G. Mendel's Law Concerning the Behavior of the Progeny of Racial Hybrids" (*Ber. deut. Bot. Ges.*, xviii, 1900, p. 158) and acknowledged the work of Mendel and Darwin in interpreting his results in accord with Mendel's law of independent assortment that demonstrated that different genes separate independently from one another during generation of reproductive cells.

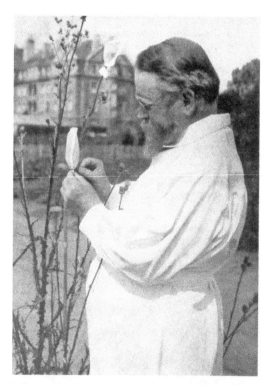

**Figure 3.7.** Karl Franz Joseph Correns (1864–1933). German botanist and geneticist who rediscovered and acknowledged the work of Mendel. Reproduced from Hans Stubbe: *Kurze Geschichte der Genetik bis zur Wiederentdeckung Gregor Mendels* Jena, 2. Auflage 1965 Quelle dort: "Photo Verlag Scherl, Berlin."

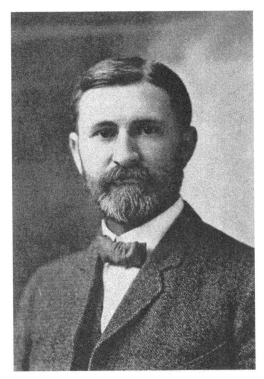

**Figure 3.8.** William Jasper Spillman (1863–1931). American agricultural economist and rediscoverer of Mendel's laws of inheritance.

William Jasper Spillman (1863–1931) (see Figure 3.8) was an American wheat geneticist and agricultural economist who wished to use genetic concepts to develop varieties of wheat that were adaptable and more suitable to the northwest United States. He was aware of Mendel's work with peas and in 1901 published his results corroborating the role of Mendelian genetic principles to wheat breeding.

Through the simultaneous but independent work of these three European botanists and one American wheat geneticist, the work and the discoveries of Mendel were rediscovered and their significance to genetics finally came to be widely known and appreciated. The rediscovery of Mendel not only opened the door to an understanding of plant genetics and principles of plant breeding but also began to exert powerful influence on the general scientific and genetics community. It is interesting that so much of this early history of genetics came from botanists and plant physiologists, but it was still to be determined if these principles of inheritance had any relevance to human biology. That application to Mendel's epochal discoveries almost half a century earlier was about to change with the work of the English physician Archibald Garrod.

# 4
# The rediscovery of Mendel, Garrod and human biochemical genetics

The uncertainty about the possible relevance of these advances in plant genetics to human biology and human disease was all to change in the first decade of the 20th century. The groundwork to this revolutionary change was being laid for an extension of Mendelian concepts to human traits, largely by William Bateson, the English evolutionist at the University of Cambridge (see Figure 4.1). Bateson was an enthusiastic popularizer of the newly rediscovered genetic concepts of Mendel, and the first person to apply the term "genetics" to the study of inheritance and the science of biological variation to explain human inherited traits.

The first person to apply these new Mendelian concepts directly to human disease was Archibald Garrod, an English physician at Great Ormond Street Hospital and St. Bartholomew's Hospital in London (see Figures 4.2 and 4.3).

Garrod was aware of Bateson's teachings and came to interpret his clinical observations in accordance with the Mendelian laws of inheritance. Garrod was studying and caring for patients suffering from several familial-inherited diseases, including alkaptonuria, pentosuria, cystinuria and albinism. He was particularly interested in the familial disease alkaptonuria that is characterized by the excretion of dark urine and by the development of arthritis apparently related to the deposit of purple-brown pigment (homogentisic acid) in cartilage and connective tissue (Figure 4.4). He described the familial pattern of inheritance of alkaptonuria in a paper, "The Incidence of Alkaptonuria: A Study of Chemical Individuality," that he published in 1902. That foundational paper not only described the Mendelian basis for the biochemical error in alkaptonuria but also clarified the Mendelian inheritance mechanisms of the three other diseases. This publication represents the birth of human chemical biology and establishes the genetic basis of human chemical biology and individuality, firmly bringing the Mendelian concepts to human disease. Noting the similarity of inheritance pattern of alkaptonuria with the several other familial diseases that he was treating—cystinuria, pentosuria and

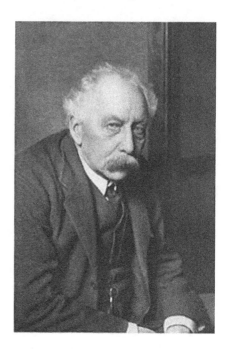

**Figure 4.1.** William Bateson (1861–1926).

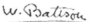

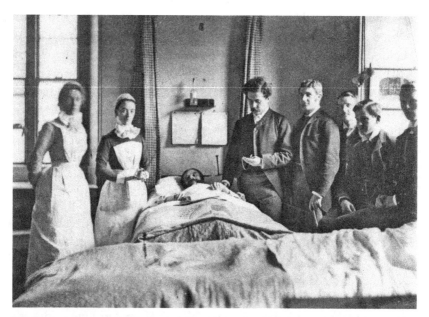

**Figure 4.2.** Sir Archibald Garrod (1857–1936). English physician and Regius Professor of Medicine at the University of Oxford who first applied Mendel's laws of genetic inheritance to human disease with his concept of chemical individuality and "inborn errors of metabolism." He is widely considered the father of chemical biology. Courtesy of Barts health NHS Trust Archives, image reference: SBHX8/956.

MENDEL, GARROD AND HUMAN BIOCHEMICAL GENETICS   33

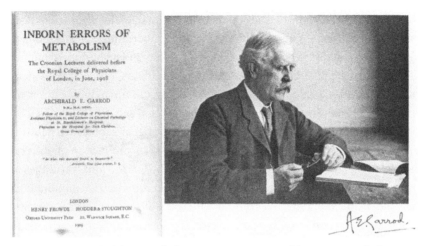

**Figure 4.3.** Archibald Garrod's famous presentation of the concept of inborn errors of metabolism in his 1908 Croonian Lectures at the Royal College of Physicians.

albinism—Garrod developed the concept of "inborn errors of metabolism," every part of which phrase is significant and which reveals Garrod's landmark intuitive understanding of human chemical biology. Garrod proved that these familial diseases are "inborn," therefore not resulting from external causes;

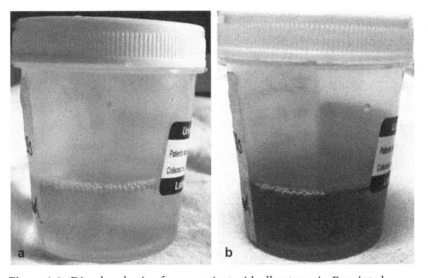

**Figure 4.4.** Discolored urine from a patient with alkaptonuria. Reprinted with permission from Vikas Sharma, Rajendra B. Nerli, Prasad V. Magdum, Abhijith Mudegoudra, Murigendra B. Hiremath, Alkaptonuria in a 6 Year Old Patient: Case Report. *Urology Case Reports*, 3/6, 2015, 188–189. https://doi.org/10.1016/j.eucr.2015.07.013.

that they are "errors" or aberrations of normal human biology; and that those errors cause disease or dysfunction by causing aberrations of metabolism. Garrod presented his epochal advancement in the understanding of human genetic disease in the Croonian Lectures to the Royal College of Physicians in London in 1908, and this represented the birth of human biochemical genetics and human chemical biology. The concept that genetically inherited biochemical defects cause disease by disrupting normal metabolic mechanisms and by blocking production of vital metabolites or by production of an aberrant toxic metabolite was an epochal discovery by Garrod and constitutes to this day much of our conceptualization of human disease. This monumental new biochemical understanding of disease was not only new understanding of disease causation but just as important, it suggested a direct new route to therapy. According to Garrod's principle of inborn errors of metabolism, effective treatment of genetic disease could be achieved by one of several independent routes—by circumventing a metabolic block and supplying a blocked metabolite to the body, by preventing production of a toxic metabolite, or ultimately by correction or reconstitution of the underlying genetic defect—i.e., "gene therapy."

Garrod's concept of "inborn errors of metabolism" described the pathogenesis of several human genetic diseases but it provided no immediate treatments for any of them. But Garrod's work certainly did predict the first rational approach to therapy for inborn errors of metabolism. The first successful treatment of a human genetic or developmental disease by the product replacement approach so well predicted by Garrod's work occurred in 1921 in the case of insulin deficiency in diabetes mellitus. At that time, the basis for the development of diabetes was not known—was it a genetic disease, was it a developmental problem, was it an infectious disease? It was only much later in the 20th century that it became clear that there are several kinds of diabetes—type I known to result from the immune destruction of pancreatic islet cells causing the impaired production of insulin by the pancreatic islet cells, and type II characterized by body-wide tissue insensitivity to insulin. The best model available to investigators at the beginning of the 20th century was essentially a model of type I diabetes that could be created by surgical removal of the pancreas. Without a source of insulin production, severe and life-threatening and often fatal diabetes resulted. In 1910, the English physiologist Edward Sharpey-Schafer identified the relevant missing product and called it "insulin" because of its production in the pancreatic islet cells of Langerhans.

In 1921, the Canadian scientist Frederick Banting and his doctoral student Charles Best applied the Mendelian principle of replacing a missing metabolic product for purposes of therapy, extracted insulin from normal pancreas tissue and injected it intravenously into pancreatectomized dogs that were showing symptoms of diabetes, leading to rapid correction of the elevated glucose levels in the blood and prevention of disease (see Figure 4.5).

While the disease model of pancreatectomized dogs was a surgical model rather than a naturally occurring inborn error of metabolism, the concept of replacing a missing metabolic product is a natural central consequence of the Garrodian concept of the causes of inborn errors of metabolism. After the success of the dog studies, the Canadian doctors proceeded to isolate insulin from cows and used it to treat a severely ill 14-year-old diabetic boy. The boy recovered and after an initial allergic reaction to the first injection,

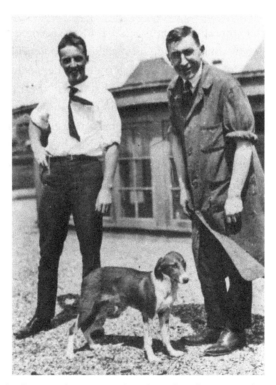

**Figure 4.5.** Charles Best (1899–1978) and Frederick Banting (1891–1941). Canadian scientists who established the therapeutic role of insulin in diabetes mellitus. Reproduced with kind permission from Thomas Fisher Rare Book Library, University of Toronto.

he went on to survive his life-threatening disease. This revolutionary advance established Garrod's therapeutic principle of "replace what is missing" and earned Banting the 1923 Nobel Prize for Physiology or Medicine for the discovery of insulin as a treatment for diabetes. Rather than including Best in the Nobel prize award, the Nobel committee cited James Macleod, director of the laboratory in which Banting and Best carried out their studies, as co-discoverer of insulin. Banting thought that the omission of Best failed to recognize Best's contribution to the discovery of insulin and vowed to donate half of his Nobel prize money to Best. Similarly, James Macleod showed his displeasure with the Nobel committee selection by sharing part of his prize with James Collip, another member of the Toronto team and a key participant in developing methods to purify insulin.

Through the work of these scientists and their discovery of insulin, it was clear that Garrod's description of inborn errors of metabolism therefore not only described the origin of disease but also pointed to a spectacularly effective approach to therapy, an approach that was to become one of the central principles for treatment of human metabolic and genetic diseases. The Garrod concept of inborn errors and determining the biochemical and enzymatic defect underlying a disease took a giant step toward the therapy of genetic disease. Because of the achievement of the discovery of insulin, the treatment of genetic disease graduated from merely identifying the enzymic defect causing a disease to attempts to treat disease by "replacing the missing metabolite." More than a century after that work, insulin remains the mainstay in the treatment of diabetes mellitus.

# 5

# Mutations are inherited by Mendel's laws and can cause disease. What are chromosomes? What elements in chromosomes cause disease?—The Sutton-Boveri chromosome theory

It was during the beginning of the 20th century when advances in cell biology and histology began to illuminate the mechanisms governing the rediscovered Mendelian laws of inheritance and to explain the mechanisms by which genetic information is transferred from one generation to the next. In 1902 and 1903, the American geneticist and biologist Walter Sutton (1877–1916) and the German Theodor Boveri (1862–1915) developed what came to be called the Sutton-Boveri chromosome theory that demonstrated that the linear structures known to exist in the nuclei of cells and termed "chromosomes" because of their colorful property of staining with basic dyes, were the carriers of the genetic information and that the paired determinants on the chromosomes behaved in accordance with Mendel's laws.

In 1905, the Danish biologist Wilhelm Johansen (1857–1927) published his work in which he coined the word "gene" for the basic unit of heredity as well as the terms genotype and phenotype to describe the full genetic makeup of an individual organism and its overall appearance.

## Thomas Hunt Morgan—description of chromosomes and role of genes

In a brilliant act of insight following the rediscovery of Mendel's laws, the American geneticist Thomas Hung Morgan (1866–1945) (Figure 5.1) brought the emerging fields of cell biology and genetics together when he

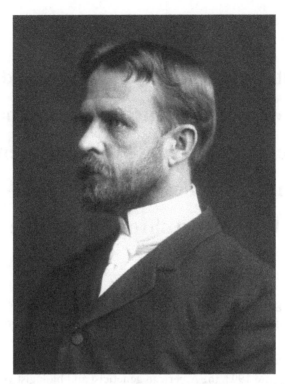

**Figure 5.1.** Thomas Hunt Morgan (1866–1945). American geneticist and evolutionary biologist who famously established the value of the *Drosophila* (fruit fly) model to elucidate chromosomal mechanisms in heredity. Reproduced from Johns Hopkins yearbook, 1891.

chose to use the fruit fly *Drosophila melanogaster* as a model system to study the mechanisms by which genetic information is transferred from one generation to another. He was aware of the de Vries concept that new species arise by sudden mutations rather than by Darwinian natural selection, and Morgan set out to use the fruit fly model to test the De Vries concept of speciation.

He established the legendary "fly room" at Columbia University, and together with a long series of brilliant students, graduate students and postdoctoral fellows, he used chemical, physical and radiation methods to create and examine thousands of *Drosophila* mutants and used the Mendelian characteristic of their inheritance patterns to discover genetic linkage and chromosomal crossing-over and to prove a model of the chromosome as a linear collection of genes like "beads on a string." They can be inherited together (linkage) or in rearranged form by exchange with other paired chromosomes (crossing-over). In 1915, Morgan and his colleagues published their epochal model of the mechanisms of genetics in *The Mechanism of Mendelian Heredity*, a book that came to be a virtual bible of genetic knowledge at that time and which proved the chromosome basis for heredity that the British biologist Conrad Waddington called "a great leap of imagination comparable with Galileo and Newton." The only thing wrong with that praise is that Morgan's work was less a product of imagination alone but far more the result of brilliant and incisive intellectual insight. That accomplishment was recognized by the award of the 1933 Nobel Prize in Medicine or Physiology and by the suggestion by the British scientist J.B.S. Haldane that the name Morgan be used to define the unit of genetic linkage. The "Morgan" is still the standard unit of genetic length learned by generations of geneticists. After Columbia, Morgan moved to the California Institute of Technology (Caltech), where he established the Division of Biology, in itself an incubator of continuing pioneering research in the 20th century.

Additional important studies of the nature of genes and the mechanisms underlying storage and transfer of genetic information came through the elegant studies by Barbara McClintock of the Cold Spring Harbor Laboratory in New York (see Figure 5.2). She worked on the unlikely system of maize

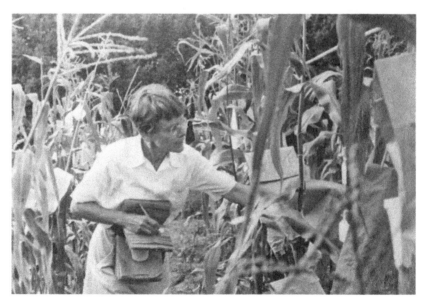

**Figure 5.2.** Barbara McClintock (1902–1992). American geneticist who elucidated the genetic map of maize and established the concept of mobile genetic elements and transposons to regulate mechanisms of gene expression. Reproduced with kind permission from the American Philosophical Society.

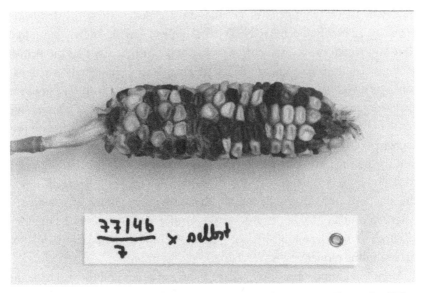

**Figure 5.3.** An ear of maize that demonstrates the phenotypic effects of mobile genetic elements in heredity. American Philosophical Society. Library. Barbara McClintock Papers. 10833. Copyright owner unknown.

genetics and wanted to understand the basis for the unstable color pattern of kernels in corn (see Figure 5.3). Her observations could not be explained by the growing traditional understanding of mutations in DNA, but rather required the explanation that maize genes are mobile in the chromosome and could transpose in response to controlling elements, thereby establishing the phenomenon of genetic transposition. Her discovery was quite heretical, and many in the genetics community were not only unconvinced but even hostile to her work. Eventually, the skeptics came to accept her extremely important findings, as did the Nobel committee for Physiology or Medicine who awarded her the Prize in 1983. From McClintock's work we learned that genes are not static or fixed in place in the chromosomes but that they can be mobile and move from place to place. It was an entirely new look at genes.

# 6
# DNA is the repository and transmitter of genetic information

By the middle of the 20th century, it had been clearly established that genetic information is transferred from one generation to another according to the laws discovered by Gregor Mendel, that errors of that transfer could lead to disease, that the normal or pathogenic information was carried and transferred by the cell bodies called "chromosomes" and more specifically by the chromosomal elements on the chromosomes called "genes" and that the genes can be transferred together as groups of "beads on a string" or in rearranged or mutated forms. But what was still entirely unknown was what it was in the gene that stored and conveyed the genetic information. What was the chemical nature of the gene, and did it have a defined structure?

The first convincing experimental answer to that puzzle came in 1928 from the work of Frederick Griffith, a bacteriologist and medical officer at the Ministry of Health in England (Figure 6.1). Research on bacterial, and especially pneumococcal infections was urgently needed at that time because of the high incidence of very serious pneumococcal infections in the 1918 influenza pandemic. Griffth studied the question of virulence of pneumococcal strains, and in classical but largely unheralded experiments known as the "Griffith Experiment," he showed that an element present in extracts of a virulent smooth (S) strain could heritably "transform" pneumococci of a nonvirulent rough (R) strain. Griffith concluded that the R strain had been heritably transformed by a component of the lethal S strain into a lethal S strain that he merely identified as TP (transforming principle).

Following on the work of Griffith in 1944, a group of scientists at the Rockefeller Institute in New York provided the first clear experimental explanation of that part of the genetic puzzle (see Figure 6.2). Oswald Avery (1877–1955) (Figure 6.3), the Canadian physician Colin MacLeod (1909–1972) (Figure 6.4), and Maclyn McCarty (1911–2005) (Figure 6.5) were trying to confirm the Griffith studies and were studying the question of what determines the rough or smooth external capsule properties of different strains of pneumococcus and if and how the properties of one strain

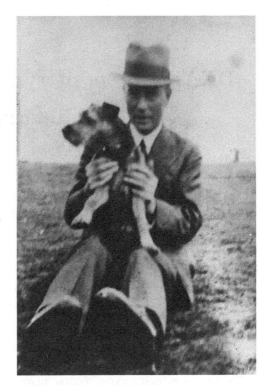

**Figure 6.1.** Frederick Griffith (1877–1941). English bacteriologist who provided the first demonstration of bacterial transformation in the famous "Griffith Experiment" and laid the groundwork for the proof that such an effect resulted from transfer of DNA from one organism to another.

can be transformed from one form to another. Avery, the leader of the Rockefeller group, was initially skeptical of Griffith's results and attributed such crucial results to possibly inadequately controlled experimental design. However, Avery and his colleagues eventually confirmed the Griffith result and identified the transforming principle as a high-molecular-weight substance that reacted positively with the Dische diphenylamine reagent. The Dische reagent was known to react with the deoxyribose moiety of DNA and not to react with RNA, protein or carbohydrate. The Avery team concluded that the agent that stored and transferred genetic information was DNA! DNA was obviously at the heart of all that science had been learning from Mendel, Garrod, Johansen, Sutton, Boveri, Morgan!

At that time, it was still completely unclear how "errors" in DNA as described by Garrod led to metabolic disruption and to disease. How did genetic defects produce aberrations in enzyme function and in altered and pathogenic cellular metabolism? Clues to that question came from work of the American geneticists George Beadle (1903–1989) (Figure 6.6) and Edward Tatum (1909–1975) (Figure 6.7), who created and studied hundreds of radiation-induced mutants of the mold *Neurospora crassa* and showed that the mutations worked

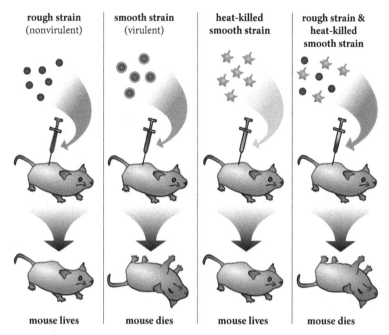

**Figure 6.2.** The "Griffith Experiment" of bacterial transformation. The studies by Frederick Griffith showed for the first time that a genetic function could be transferred from one organism to another (genetic transformation). Griffith exposed mice to a rough, non-lethal strain of pneumococcus (small dots, left panel), all mice survived. When mice were exposed to a smooth virulent strain of pneumococcus (larger dots, second panel from left), all died. Mice exposed to heat-killed smooth strain pneumococci (third panel from left) also all survived. However, mice exposed to a mixture of non-virulent rough pneumococci and heat-killed smooth virulent pneumococci all died (right panel). The previously non-virulent strain had been genetically "transformed". Griffith's work proved for the first time that genetically determined functions could be changed by an exogenous factor - i.e., "genetic transformation". This discovery is the conceptual basis for the modern field of genetic therapies. ©Madeleine Price Ball, reproduced under Creative Commons CC0 1.0 Universal Public Domain Dedication.

through the production of enzymes with defects in specific steps in amino acid metabolism, a definitive confirmation of the presumed enzymatic mechanisms underlying Garrod's "inborn errors of metabolism."

Further definitive molecular confirmation of this initial identification of DNA as the repository and transmitter of genetic information was provided in 1952 by experiments carried out at the Carnegie Institution laboratory of the Cold Spring Harbor laboratory by Alfred Hershey

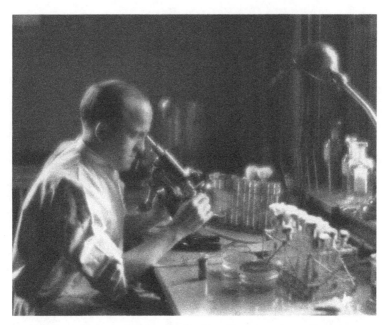

**Figure 6.3.** Oswald Avery (1877–1955). Canadian-American physician at the Rockefeller Institute in New York whose work established DNA as the repository and transmitter of genetic information. Reproduced with permission from Universal History Archive/Universal Images Group Collection.

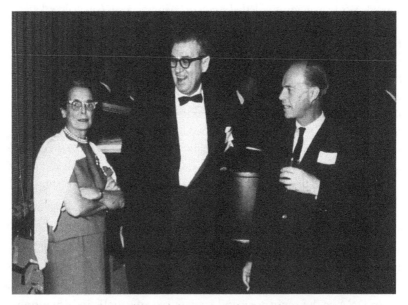

**Figure 6.4.** Colin McLeod (right) (1909–1972). Canadian-American geneticists working with his colleagues at the Rockefeller Institute in New York who discovered that the transforming principle in the "Griffith Experiment" was DNA and it was DNA that stored and transmitted genetic information from one generation to another. Courtesy of National Library of Medicine

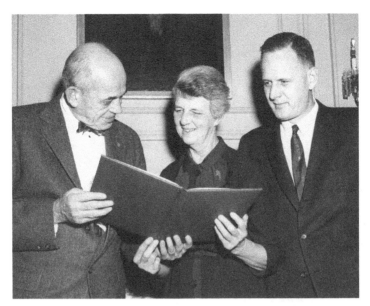

**Figure 6.5.** Maclyn McCarty (right), a member of the Avery-McLeod team from the Rockefeller Institute that proved the DNA is the macromolecule that stores and transmits genetic information. Reproduced with permission from the Smithsonian Institution Archives, Image #SIA2008-5069.

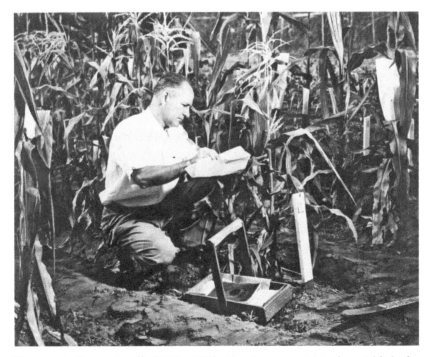

**Figure 6.6.** George Beadle (1903–1989). American geneticist who established the mechanisms by which genes regulate biochemical processes in cells. Image courtesy of Hanna Holborn Gray Special Collections Research Center, University of Chicago Library.

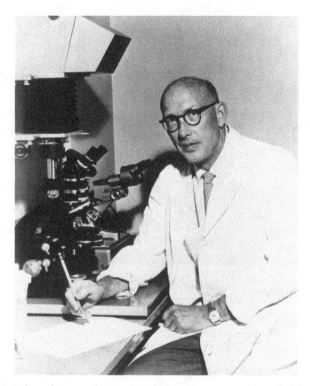

**Figure 6.7.** Edward Tatum (1909–1975). American geneticist who elucidated biochemical mechanisms of gene expression. Reproduced from U.S. National Library of Medicine, Images from the History of Medicine Collection (IHM). Photographer Unknown.

(1908–1997) (Figure 6.8) and Martha Chase (1927–2003) (Figure 6.9). These experiments quickly caught the attention of the genetics community, partly because they occurred in the midst of increasing interest at the time in phage genetics. It was well known that one of these bacterial viruses, the DNA phage T2, infected bacterial cells by attaching to the bacterial cell membrane and injecting the hereditary material into the bacterium, leading to infection and viral replication. It was uncertain exactly what that material was.

Hershey and Chase used the T2 bacteriophage labeled with 35S protein and 32P DNA to infect *E. coli* bacterial cells and followed the distribution of the radioactive labels in the cells. They showed that it was the DNA component of the virus and not the protein that was stably transferred into the infected *E. coli*, and that it was only the DNA that could be responsible for the subsequent viral replication. This discovery was the molecular genetic

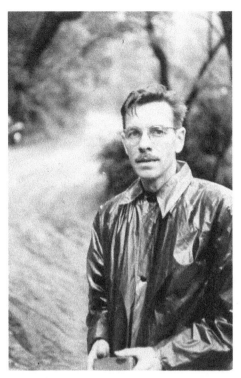

**Figure 6.8.** Alfred Hershey (1908–1997). American geneticist and bacteriologist who used a bacteriophage system to demonstrate that it was DNA and not other macromolecules such as protein that determined genetic transformation. Courtesy of Cold Spring Harbor Laboratory Archives, New York.

proof of the central role of DNA in the transmission of genetic information and earned Alfred Hershey the 1969 Nobel Prize in Medicine or Physiology. Sadly, Martha Chase did not share the prize.

The studies of Griffith, Avery and his team, and Hershey and Chase established for certain that the molecule that carries, stores and transmits genetic information is DNA. What remained glaringly unknown by the early 1950s was clarification of the mechanisms by which DNA performs those functions. At that time, a great deal was coming to be understood about DNA—especially its biochemical properties and some aspects of its structure. Most notably, the Austrian-American biochemist Erwin Chargaff (1905–2002) had famously shown in 1950 in his "Chargaff rules" that DNA always contained equal amounts of two of its four base components—adenine (A) and thymidine (T) and similarly, equal amount of the other two components cytosine (C) and guanine (G). The implications of that

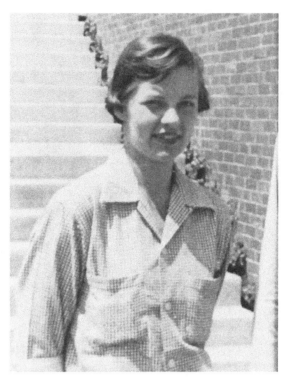

**Figure 6.9.** Martha Chase (1927–2003). American geneticist working as a student with Alfred Hershey at the Cold Spring Harbor in New York who demonstrated the role of DNA in phage infection of bacteria. Reproduced with permission from Science Photo Library.

important finding were not fully translated by Chargaff into a structural understanding of DNA. He and others at the time conjectured that the equivalency of those bases suggested that they pair along the linear DNA molecule and that they were somehow responsible for determining all of the functions of DNA through interactions with proteins. The secret of DNA would surely lie in its structure.

In 1953, together with his Caltech colleague Robert Corey (1897–1971), Linus Pauling published a paper proposing, famously and incorrectly, a triple helical structure for DNA. Pauling was famous for elucidating the three-dimensional alpha helical structure of protein, and so his work on DNA carried great weight and was potentially of immense importance. Sadly, the proposed structure was incorrect. The DNA structure the paper proposed—a triple helical structure of DNA—did not clearly explain the significance of the base composition described by Chargaff or the coding mechanism inherent in the base composition of DNA.

The Corey-Pauling paper was written in 1952 and published in 1953 shortly before the explosive paper by James Watson and Francis Crick in 1953 that described correctly the double helical structure of DNA. Any remaining mystery about the role of DNA in genetic coding and transmission was emphatically resolved with the discovery of the structure of DNA by the British crystallographer Rosalind Franklin (1920–1958) (Figure 6.10), the physicist Francis Crick (1916–2004), the geneticist James Watson (b. 1928) and the British crystallographer Maurice Wilkins (1916–2004) (Figure 6.11) and was announced to the world by Watson and Crick in their explosive publication in 1953 of the double helical

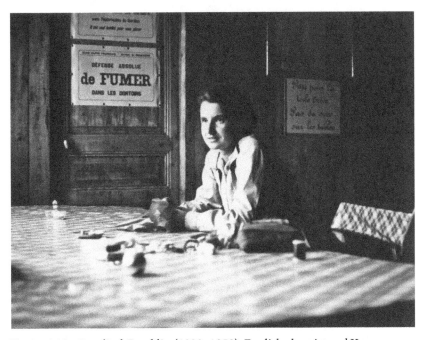

**Figure 6.10.** Rosalind Franklin (1920–1958). English chemist and X-ray crystallographer whose images of DNA were used by James Watson and Francis Crick in a somewhat controversial collaboration omitting Franklin to elucidate the double helical structure of DNA. Reproduced with permission © National Portrait Gallery, London.

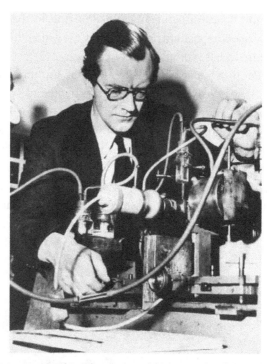

**Figure 6.11.** Maurice Wilkins (1916–2004). New Zealand. British biophysicist and X-ray crystallographer who developed instrumentation for X-ray diffraction structural studies of DNA. Reproduced from National Institutes of Health.

structure of DNA. The model was very quickly constructed and published with unheard-of speed within a month of its submission to the journal *Nature* in April 1953. The brilliance of the model took advantage of a correct structural interpretation of the Chargaff rules of base equivalency and the availability of the foundational X-ray crystallographic studies of Rosalind Franklin, a contribution that went largely uncredited by Watson and Crick in their paper, with the exception of thanks to her for "discussions." In a stroke of brilliant insight, Watson and Crick concluded that it was the specific sequence of bases on a DNA molecule that contains the genetical information for storing genetic information and for replication, although the model didn't immediately demonstrate how that information was converted into aberrant biological function (Figure 6.12). That was to become revealed in the coming decades by the birth of molecular biology.

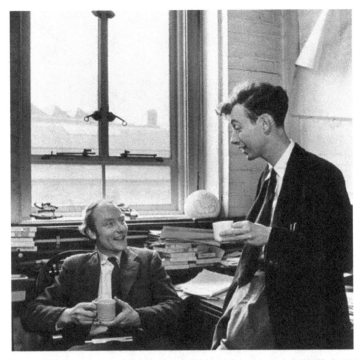

**Figure 6.12.** James Watson (right) (b. 1928) and Francis Crick (left) (1916–2004) in their office at the Molecular Biology Laboratory in Cambridge, England, ca. 1953. Molecular biologists and co-discoverers of the double helical structure of DNA. Reproduced with permission from A. Barrington Brown/ Science Source.

The crystal structure of DNA in itself could not immediately identify the mechanisms by which it encoded the genetic information. That breakthrough came with the discovery by Crick and his colleagues in 1961 of the triplet nature of the genetic code and the following "cracking the genetic code" in 1965 by the American Marshall Nirenberg (1927–2010) and his German postdoctoral fellow Heinrich Matthaei at the U.S National Institutes of Health. Nirenberg and Matthaei showed that when they used a protein-synthesizing extract containing all of the component unlabeled amino acids and radioactive phenylalanine, only the extract to which they had also added synthetic poly-uracil RNA produced radioactively labeled polypeptide (see Figure 6.13). A string of uracil bases encodes the amino acid phenylalanine! Similar experiments then identified the triplet RNA code for the rest of the amino acids.

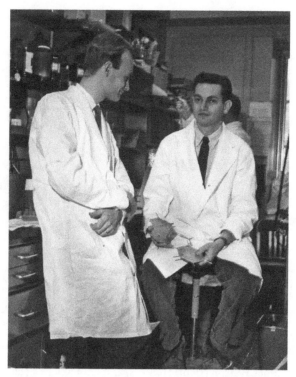

**Figure 6.13.** Heinrich Matthaei (left) (b. 1929) and Marshall Nirenberg (right) (1927–2010). Geneticists and biochemists at the U.S. National Institutes of Health who demonstrated the role of RNA in mechanisms by which DNA directed the production of polypeptides. This was an experimental demonstration of the molecular role of messenger RNA. Reproduced with permission from MacVicar, N., National Institute of Health (U.S.) The Marshall W. Nirenberg Papers (Profiles in Science).

Their discovery combined with the mechanisms discovered by the chemists Robert Holley and Gobind Khorana to explain how the base triplets specified interaction with "transfer RNAs" to deliver amino acids to ribosomes, the protein-synthesizing machinery of the cells.

# 7

# From inborn errors to molecular disease

With the advances during the 20th century in the science of cellular biochemistry and its role in human disease, it was becoming clear that Garrod's concept of inborn errors of metabolism could not be restricted to the rare, nonlethal diseases studied by Garrod, but rather that many and possibly most human diseases, common or rare, lethal or benign, should be seen to be caused by, or at least partly due to, genetic defects. During most of the mid- and late-20th century, the biochemical and metabolic bases for hundreds of human diseases were discovered, which facilitated the discovery of drug-based approaches to treatment. A now-classic example of this biochemical approach to understanding and treating a genetic disease came in the case of the disease familial hypercholesterolemia, in which elucidation of the metabolic defects of cholesterol metabolism responsible for the disease led to subsequent discovery of effective and life-saving drug-based therapies for this lethal disease and, in later years, led to the enormously popular and life-saving drug-based treatment of hypercholesterolemia with "statins." This work demonstrated that successful therapy of a genetic disease could take place by manipulation of the associated biochemical and metabolic defects. Fix the broken metabolism just as in the case of insulin and diabetes! (Figure 7.1)

But of course, the understanding of the genetic basis for human disease progressed and accelerated during the decades following Garrod's description of "inborn errors of metabolism," as knowledge was growing about genetics and its role in the development of human disease along with a parallel revolution in the understanding of proteins, their structure and their role in disease. Linus Pauling (Figure 7.2), the Caltech chemist and physicist most renowned for his work on the nature of the chemical bond, the development of X-ray crystallographic methods for examining protein structure and his fervent anti-nuclear war activism, applied his expertise in protein chemistry to examine the hemoglobin protein from normal individuals and from patients with sickle cell anemia and from normal carriers of the sickle cell trait (see Figure 7.3). In 1949, Pauling and his colleagues Harvey Itano,

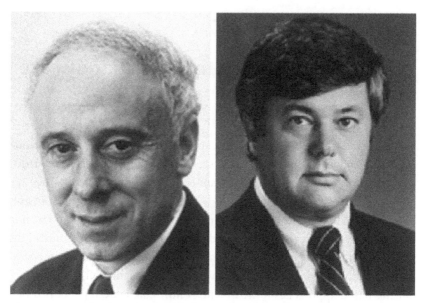

**Figure 7.1.** Michael Brown (right) (b. 1941) and Joseph Goldstein (left) (b. 1940). American physicians and geneticists who discovered the low-density lipoprotein receptor and its role in regulating cholesterol metabolism. Their studies established the mechanisms underlying genetic disease and pointed to effective methods of therapy. Reproduced with permission from: Raju, Tonse NK. The Nobel Chronicles. *The Lancet.* Volume 355, Issue 9201, P416. © Elsevier 2000.

John Singer and Ibert Wells reported that the hemoglobin protein from these groups showed differences in mobility in an electrical field, and they coined the term "molecular disease" to underscore for the first time that a human genetic disease was proven to result from expression of aberrant structure and abnormal function of the encoded protein (see Figure 7.4). Of course, there was much still to be determined, especially the question of how many amino acids were altered in the sickle protein.

Newly armed with this concept of molecular disease and the evidence that the sickle cell hemoglobin (Hb-S) presented an ideal opportunity to understand how an aberrant protein causes disease, the German-American chemist Vernon Ingram (1924–2006) took advantage of the many advances in protein characterization to identify precisely, for the first time, the mechanism by which a mutant gene causes production of an aberrantly functioning protein.

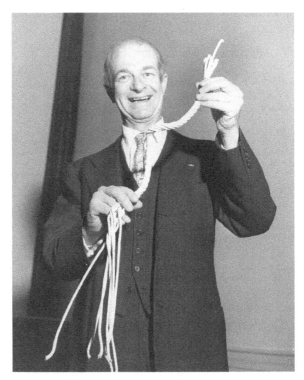

**Figure 7.2.** Linus Pauling (1901–1994). American theoretical and structural chemist, two-time Nobel Prize winner and peace activist, using a twisted length of rope to illustrate a proposed helical structure of DNA. Reproduced from Smithsonian Institution Acc. 90-105 - Science Service, Records, 1920s–1970s.

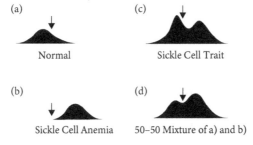

**Figure 7.3.** Demonstration of aberrant electrophoretic mobility of beta globin from patients with sickle cell anemia. The sickle protein migrated to a different position in the electric field, proving a structural alteration is the basis for its altered properties. This demonstration established the concept of "molecular disease". Reproduced with permission from 1949. L. Pauling, H. Itano et al. Sickle Cell Anemia, a Molecular Disease. *Science* 110: 543–548. © AAAS.

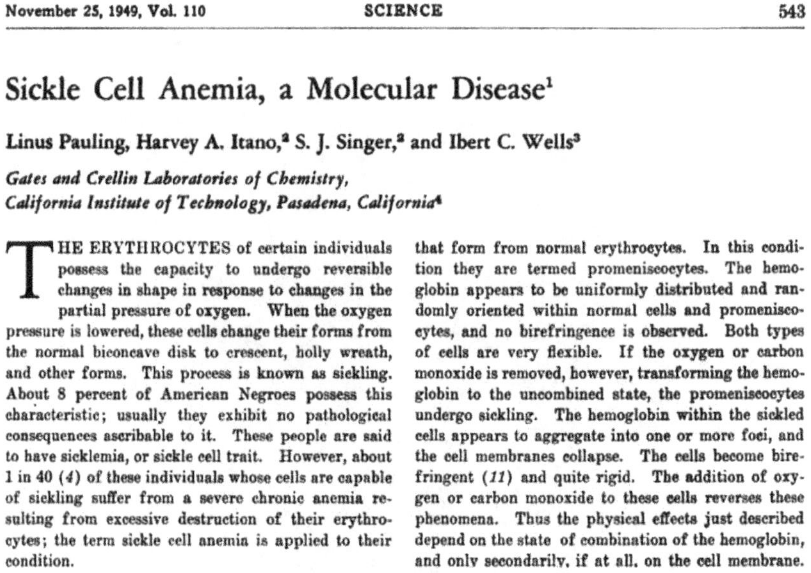

## Sickle Cell Anemia, a Molecular Disease[1]

Linus Pauling, Harvey A. Itano,[2] S. J. Singer,[2] and Ibert C. Wells[3]

*Gates and Crellin Laboratories of Chemistry,*
*California Institute of Technology, Pasadena, California*[4]

THE ERYTHROCYTES of certain individuals possess the capacity to undergo reversible changes in shape in response to changes in the partial pressure of oxygen. When the oxygen pressure is lowered, these cells change their forms from the normal biconcave disk to crescent, holly wreath, and other forms. This process is known as sickling. About 8 percent of American Negroes possess this characteristic; usually they exhibit no pathological consequences ascribable to it. These people are said to have sicklemia, or sickle cell trait. However, about 1 in 40 (4) of these individuals whose cells are capable of sickling suffer from a severe chronic anemia resulting from excessive destruction of their erythrocytes; the term sickle cell anemia is applied to their condition. that form from normal erythrocytes. In this condition they are termed promeniscocytes. The hemoglobin appears to be uniformly distributed and randomly oriented within normal cells and promeniscocytes, and no birefringence is observed. Both types of cells are very flexible. If the oxygen or carbon monoxide is removed, however, transforming the hemoglobin to the uncombined state, the promeniscocytes undergo sickling. The hemoglobin within the sickled cells appears to aggregate into one or more foci, and the cell membranes collapse. The cells become birefringent (11) and quite rigid. The addition of oxygen or carbon monoxide to these cells reverses these phenomena. Thus the physical effects just described depend on the state of combination of the hemoglobin, and only secondarily, if at all, on the cell membrane.

Figure 7.4. Publication by Pauling and his colleagues using their results with the structure of sickle cell hemoglobin to establish the concept of "molecular disease." Reproduced with permission from 1949. L. Pauling, H. Itano et al. Sickle Cell Anemia, a Molecular Disease. *Science* 110: 543–548. © AAAS.

Vernon Ingram was working at the Medical Research Council Laboratory of Molecular Biology (LMB) in Cambridge, England, where the Viennese crystallographer Max Perutz had assembled a group of protein crystallographers to determine the structure of proteins, particularly the hemoglobin molecular, and where Frederick Sanger was developing his foundational methods to characterize protein structure in order to determine their amino acid makeup and, especially, to deduce their sequence (see Figure 7.5). His work put a final nail in the coffin of the idea that proteins were possibly just disordered clumps of amino acids but were, in fact, composed of a specific linear sequence of amino acids in a defined and reproducible sequence. The LMB was the ideal laboratory for Ingram to examine the structural abnormality of Hb-S and why and how the mutation in Hb-S deformed the red blood cells and caused them to clog the small blood vessels and cause disease. Indeed, with all of the brilliant protein-characterizing technology of the Laboratory of Molecular Biology of the Medical Research Council behind him, Ingram showed in 1956 that the Hb-S protein displayed a single amino acid change—substitution of glutamic acid at position 6 with valine—and that small change caused the debilitating and even lethal disease

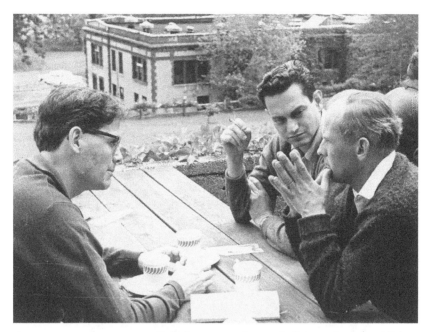

**Figure 7.5.** Vernon Ingram (left) (1924–2006), Marshall Nirenberg (middle) (1927–2010) and Matthias Staehelin (right) at the 1963 Cold Spring Harbor Symposium on Synthesis and Structure of Macromolecules. Courtesy of Cold Spring Harbor Laboratory Archives, New York.

sickle cell anemia. Ingram had proven that the effect of a simple Mendelian change can cause substitution of a single amino acid and thereby cause severe genetic disease.

These discoveries by Pauling and Ingram and their colleagues demonstrated that genetic defects cause clinical disease by altering the structure and function of the enzymes or other protein gene products, a finding that extended the purely electrophoretic changes demonstrated by Pauling and thereby finally provided a molecular explanation Garrod's "inborn errors of metabolism."

These advances in molecular and human genetics by Pauling and Ingram produced a far greater understanding of human clinical genetics and of the pathogenesis and the role of aberrant genetic mechanisms in human disease. During the middle-20th century, many additional advances in biochemistry and medical genetics identified the genetic defects and the resulting biochemical and metabolic aberrations in many human diseases. Beginning in 1966, the geneticist Victor McKusick at Johns Hopkins University catalogued the known Mendelian diseases in a landmark publication known as *Mendelian Inheritance in Man* (MIM) (Figures 7.6 and 7.7).

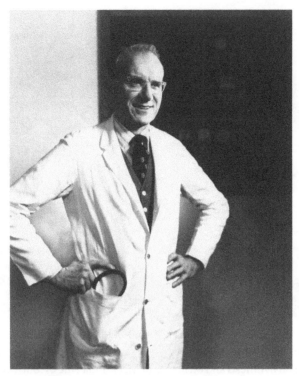

**Figure 7.6.** Victor McKusick (1921–2008). Often referred to as the "father of medical genetics" for his establishment of the compilation in the *Mendelian Inheritance in Man* and its characterization of human genetic disease. © Yousuf Karsh.

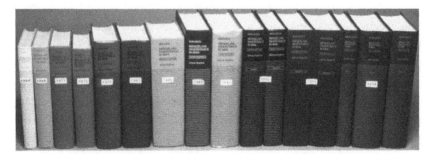

**Figure 7.7.** The growth of human genetics in the latter part of the 20th century as illustrated by the editions of the print version of McKusick's *Mendelian Inheritance in Man*. From 1966 to 1998. Reproduced with permission from McKusick, Victor A. Mendelian Inheritance In Man, OMIM. *Perspectives In Human Genetics*, Volume 80, Issue 4, P588–604. © 2007 The American Society of Human Genetics. Published by Elsevier Inc.

The first edition of MIM in 1966 described the phenotypes of 1486 human genetic disorders. Over the following years until 1998, twelve print editions appeared, documenting the explosive growth in human clinical genetics. The size of the print volumes dramatically illustrated the growth of human clinical genetics during those three decades. The first edition was a thin, single volume of 1486 diseases entries, while the twelfth edition is a large, three-volume set containing 9,000 disease entries and genomic map information on 4,000 genes and identifying the precise point mutations known to cause 700 genetic diseases and cancers.

To keep up with the increase in knowledge of genetic disease and to take advantage of internet-based computerized record-keeping, online editions (Online Mendelian Inheritance in Man—OMIM) were created by the Welch Medical Library at Johns Hopkins in 1987 and rapidly became a valuable worldwide genetics resource (Figure 7.8). The expansion of knowledge and

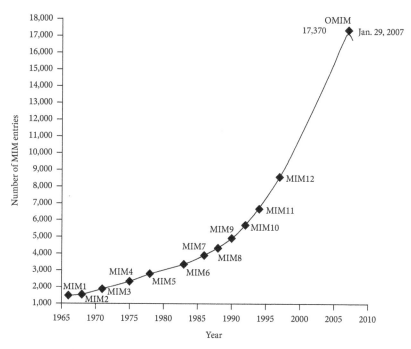

**Figure 7.8.** The explosive growth of the number of recognized human genetic diseases listed in the print and online versions of McKusick's *Mendelian Inheritance in Man*. Reproduced with permission from McKusick, Victor A. Mendelian Inheritance In Man, OMIM. *Perspectives In Human Genetics*, Volume 80, Issue 4, P588–604. © 2007 The American Society of Human Genetics. Published by Elsevier Inc.

human genetic disease was further catalyzed in 1995 by the National Library of Medicine. In constructing this compendium—now well into its more than half-century history—McKusick established his unique role as the single most important early shepherd of human clinical genetics data. His MIM and OMIM presented the almost entirely descriptive terrain of genetics which made available a remarkable goldmine of human disease models that were obviously ripe for attempts at genetic correction (i.e., gene therapy). That enormous advance brought on a new era of a more manipulative role for genetics as would be needed to not merely understand disease but also to create the conceptually new form of disease treatment (i.e., gene therapy).

# 8
# First faltering steps toward gene therapy— viruses as gene transfer vectors

By the middle of the 1960s, the air was becoming thick with the idea that the exploding knowledge of genetics not only allowed an understanding of the mechanisms of genetic disease but also potentially made obvious the creation of definitive new approaches to treatment through genetic modification of human genomes to circumvent disease-related genes. A variety of viruses emerged as candidates for introducing potentially therapeutic wild-type genes into genetically defective cells. Gene transfer, because it had become clear that the job description of viruses, whether they be bacterial viruses (phages) or mammalian viruses, is precisely the stable, efficient and heritable transfer of genes into cells.

The Hershey-Chase experiment took advantage of that viral property of efficient gene transfer to prove that DNA was the material that many viruses use to transfer genetic information into host cells. Similarly, the studies of Dulbecco and his colleagues in the early to mid-1960s demonstrated that the mammalian papova viruses (papilloma-polyoma-SV40) transferred a tumorigenic gene into mammalian cells with the resulting transformation of the normal cell into a cancer-producing cell.

If methods could be developed to copy those viral mechanisms and to remove the pathogenic functions of viruses and replace them with therapeutic genes, that would be exactly the technique required to convert pathogenic mammalian viruses into gene transfer agents to allow new kinds of studies of viral and mammalian genetics. Those were exciting possibilities to virologists and geneticists because they implied that the same property of mammalian viruses might be used to develop extremely efficient methods to introduce therapeutic genes into humans suffering from inborn errors and possibly even other gene-related diseases—i.e., "gene therapy."

Among the very earliest virologists trying to capitalize on those new concepts were the virologists Stanfield Rogers and Peter Pfuderer at the U.S. Oak Ridge National Laboratory, who wished to develop methods to chemically modify a viral genome to change its transducing properties, as reported in a *Nature* paper in 1968. The Rogers team added poly(A) tails to the genome of tobacco mosaic virus (TMV), and tobacco leaves infected with the chemically modified TMV virus demonstrated elevated levels of tetra-lysine and penta-lysine oligomers, indicating that the altered TMV genome was expressed.

This finding was intriguing to virologists and geneticists and seemed to point to a method of constructing transducing viruses for potential application to human disease therapy. The approach was certainly imaginative and farsighted but premature, partly because it preceded the advent of the recombinant DNA techniques. The entirely chemical approach to constructing a gene transferring virus vector for mammalian and even human application came to be replaced by more efficient methods for virus vector design that were enabled by recombinant DNA techniques.

Rogers proceeded to use a naturally occurring virus for the first attempt at gene therapy in humans. It had previously been observed that some people who had worked with the well-known Shope papilloma virus showed decreased serum levels of the amino acid arginine. Rogers assumed incorrectly and without experimental evidence that the virus genome encoded an arginase gene and that infection with the virus might lead to expression of the viral arginase gene and therefore might correct the genetic defect in arginase-deficient patients.

In 1958, he and his colleagues at the Oak Ridge National laboratory in Tennessee proposed that the genome of the Shope papilloma virus that was responsible for warts in rabbits might include an arginase gene and that the intact naturally occurring virus might therefore be used to transfer a functional arginase gene into several young children in Germany whom he had been made aware of and who were suffering from the extremely rare neurological disease hyperargininemia, an inborn error of arginine metabolism deficiency that causes severe growth problems, seizures, failure to thrive and intellectual delay.

Rogers and his German clinical colleague Dr. H.G. Terheggen proceeded to inoculate the three young German arginase-deficient children with the Shope virus. The concept was flawed because there was no experimental evidence that the Shope virus genome encoded an arginase gene, even though there was some biochemical evidence that infection with the Shope virus could induce expression of an arginase activity that resembled cellular arginase. Nevertheless, as interesting as the concept was of using a naturally occurring virus to carry a potentially therapeutic gene, in 1975 Terheggen reported that the study had failed to decrease arginine levels in the children or to alleviate their symptoms. Terheggen surmised without evidence that the reason for the failure might have been that the virus had been overly purified. But it was later established that the genome of Shope virus does not encode an arginase function.*

In the middle 1960s, Renato Dulbecco and his group at the Salk Institute in La Jolla, California, made the important and exciting discovery that the tumor viruses polyoma and SV40 transformed normal cells into tumor cells by transferring one of their genes into the cells and that the resulting cells were no longer able to obey cellular signals to stop replicating in a normal controlled way. Those results not only revolutionized cancer research but also raised the possibility that these and possibly other viruses might be genetically modified and tamed to carry potentially therapeutic genes rather than harmful cancer-causing genes into cells.

In the late 1960s and early 1970, several groups began to examine the use of these viruses to test their potential use for transferring foreign genetic material information into mammalian cells for the purpose of therapy. The idea was to "disarm" a pathogenic virus and to use its residual capability of efficient gene transfer as a means of introducing therapeutic genetic material into diseased tissues. It is a modern restatement of the Old Testament judgement the virtuous "shall beat their swords into plowshares" (Isaiah 2:4) (see Figure 8.1).

Early in that period, tools for recombinant DNA had not yet become available, and virologists did not know how to create genetically modified viral genomes, but alternative concepts emerged for taking advantage of these efficient gene transfer agents in a setting of potential gene therapy.

During my time in Dulbecco's laboratory in 1968, my goal was to build suitable gene-transferring derivatives of polyoma virus. The concept was to take preparations of purified polyoma virus, chemically disaggregate the virus particles and then force them to reassemble in vitro in the presence of foreign DNA, thereby constructing "pseudoviruses" artificially packaged with nonviral DNA. I succeeded in disaggregating and reassembling virus-like DNA–protein complexes and even virus-like particles in cell-free conditions in vitro, but not in encapsidating detectable amounts of foreign DNA.

---

* Use of Viruses as Carriers of Added Genetic Information. Stanfield Rogers & Peter Pfuderer. *Nature* 219, 749–751 (17 August 1968). doi:10.1038/219749a0.

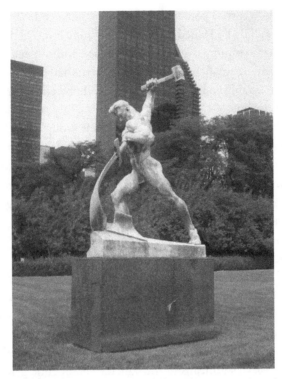

**Figure 8.1.** Statue "Swords into Plowshares" by Yeygeny Vuchetich in the garden of the United Nations in New York City. It is a convincing artistic depiction of the modification of a tool for harm into a tool for good, the underlying concept of converting a pathogenic virus into a genetic therapeutic agent. Courtesy of Rodsan18.

About the same time, Vasken Aposhian, a toxicologist at the University of Arizona, and his colleagues envisioned the use of polyoma "pseudoviruses," viral capsids that had packaged cellular DNA rather than viral DNA, to constitute a transducing virus agent carrying foreign and potentially therapeutic DNA suitable for "gene therapy." In 1971, he and his colleagues reported that they had shown some transfer into infected cells of the nonviral cellular DNA carried by polyoma pseudovirions, but they did not demonstrate expression or biological function of the foreign genetic material.

In studies similar to those that I carried out in the Dulbecco laboratory, Aposhian showed in 1980 that empty polyoma particles could indeed encapsidate polyoma DNA in a cell-free in vitro system. As with my studies on in vitro–assembled virus-like particles, the approach could not include methods to package the pseudovirus particles with potentially therapeutic genes, because the recombinant DNA tools needed for that approach were not yet available.

Those early approaches to using papova virus pseudovirions for gene transfer into host cells seemed a dead end as far as application in gene therapy approaches was concerned. The papova virus approach gave way to more effective and more efficient viral gene transfer approaches, especially those involved in murine retroviruses, adenoviruses and adeno-associated viruses. They might have proven more productive if the DNA for in vitro packaging had consisted of cloned genes rather than bulk cellular DNA, but the recombinant DNA technology for cloning and purifying genes was not to come until the early 1970s.

# 9

# Birth of molecular biology and recombinant DNA—the remarkable 1960s-1970s

The decades of the 1950s-1970s witnessed the unprecedented explosion of knowledge and technology of genetics and of the role of DNA in storing and transmitting genetic information. Principal advances included the description by the American biochemist Arthur Kornberg (1918-2007) (Figure 9.1) and the Spanish physician and biochemist Severo Ochoa (1905-1993) (Figure 9.2) of the enzymological mechanisms of nucleic acid biosynthesis, including Kornberg's isolation of the first enzyme known to drive DNA biosynthesis—DNA polymerase I. These studies were vital in laying the groundwork for much of the progress during the following several decades in characterizing the biochemical mechanisms of cellular function and replication.

That progress, a truly golden age of biology, was the effort of many laboratories through the scientific world, but without doubt much of it was driven by the improbable confluence of scientific brilliance at a small number of major scientific meccas including the Pasteur Institute in Paris, the Medical Research Council of the U.K. Laboratory of Molecular Biology (LMB) in Cambridge, England, and the U.S. National Institutes of Health and Stanford University. As if overnight, the mechanisms determining the flow of genetic information from DNA to protein came to be understood. In 1961, an intermediary RNA molecule in that flow of information (called "messenger RNA") was proposed and discovered by Francois Jacob and Jacques Monod (Figure 9.3) of the Pasteur Institute in Paris, and more or less simultaneously by Crick and Sydney Brenner (1927-2019) (Figure 9.4) and their colleagues at the Cambridge LMB laboratory.

The description of an intermediary "messenger RNA" solidified the concept, originally proposed by Francis Crick (Figure 9.5), that genetic information flows by a process of "transcription" from DNA to the intermediary

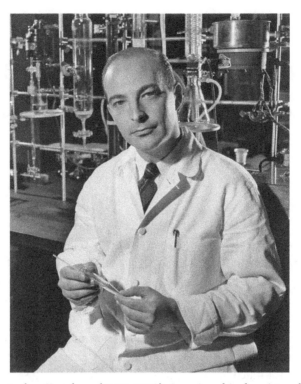

**Figure 9.1.** Arthur Kornberg (1918–2007). American biochemist and winner with the Spanish physician and biochemist Severo Ochoa of the 1959 Nobel Prize in Physiology or Medicine for his studies of the mechanisms of RNA and DNA biosynthesis. Reproduced from National Institutes of Health.

"messenger" RNA and then "translation" to the functional genetic end product, protein, but never back from protein to DNA or RNA. This central dogma concept states that genetic information never flows backward from protein to DNA (Figure 9.6).

With the birth of molecular biology and the rapidly expanding understanding of genetics and of the flow of genetic information came the explosive emergence in the early 1970s of recombinant DNA technology and gene isolation. The tools provided by the new knowledge of how genetic information is stored and transmitted and how it is expressed and controlled became immensely powerful new methods for designing and manipulating the genetic machinery of the cell, possibly even for treatment of human genetic disease. Early clues for how this might be accomplished came from the laboratory of Renato Dulbecco (Figure 9.7) at the Salk Institute in La Jolla,

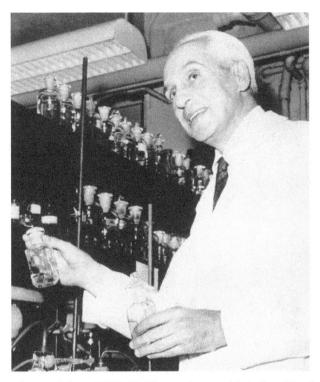

Figure 9.2. Severo Ochoa (1905–1993), co-winner with Arthur Kornberg of the 1959 Nobel Prize in Physiology or Medicine.

California, who had just discovered that the DNA tumor viruses SV40 and polyoma brought about tumorigenic changes in infected mammalian cells by introducing a foreign gene—in this case a viral transforming gene—into the infected cell genome in a heritable and expressed form. The inescapable conclusion from these results was that some kinds of viruses held the secret to how to transfer functional and potentially therapeutic foreign genetic material into mammalian cells.

My postdoctoral colleague Richard Roblin (Figure 9.8) in the Dulbecco laboratory and I recognized the potential application of this knowledge to human disease. In 1972, we proposed that gene-base therapies would be inevitable and even appropriate that the exploding genetic and virology technology would and should be applied to the treatment human genetic disease through the use of gene transferring viruses, as suggested by the Dulbecco discoveries. But just how such a proposed transfer of genetic information could be carried out for treatment of human disease was not at all

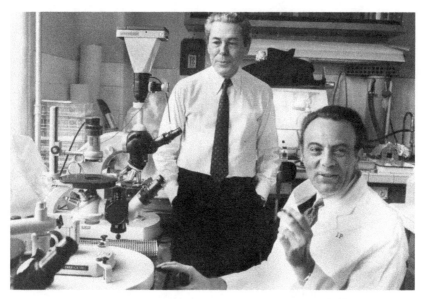

**Figure 9.3.** Jacques Monod (left) (1910–1976) and Francois Jacob (right) (1920–2013). Principal founders of modern molecular biology through their groundbreaking studies of mechanisms of gene expression and regulation, including some of the earliest studies identifying messenger RNA. Monod was active with the French Resistance during the Nazi occupation, becoming chief of staff of the French Forces of the Interior. Jacob served with the French army in the African campaign and was seriously injured. Monod and Jacob shared the 1965 Nobel Prize in Physiology or Medicine with their Pasteur Institute colleague Andre Lwoff. Reproduced from © AGIP/Bridgeman Images.

evident—which viruses? How could such agents be produced? (Figure 9.9). Our intuition an should not have come as a great surprise, since it is precisely the job description of viruses to introduce foreign genetic information in target cells. Our published proposal for text has been edited to present therapeutic for gene transferring viruses became a foundational paper in gene therapy (Figure 9.10).

Critical advances to solve those problems burst on the scene in the following epochal era of the 1970s that permitted isolation and characterization of normal and disease-related genes. These stunning advances included the discovery and use of restriction enzymes, reverse transcriptase and methods to construct viral gene transfer agents.

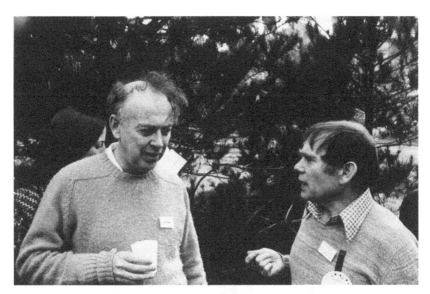

**Figure 9.4.** Sydney Brenner (right) (1927–2019) with James Watson (left) at the Cold Spring Harbor in New York. Brenner was a South African–British scientist and central figure in many of the advances in molecular biology from his base in the cauldron of scientific discovery at the Molecular Biology Laboratory in Cambridge, England, including the concept and the experimental demonstration of messenger RNA. He received the 2002 Nobel Prize in Physiology or Medicine. Reproduced from National Institutes of Health.

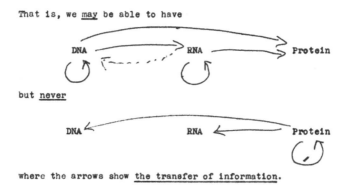

**Figure 9.5.** A diagram from a presentation by Francis Crick of the "central dogma of molecular biology"—the concept that genetic information flows from DNA to RNA to protein but never back from protein to DNA or RNA. Reproduced from Wellcome Library for the History of Understanding of Medicine. Francis Harry Compton Crick Papers.

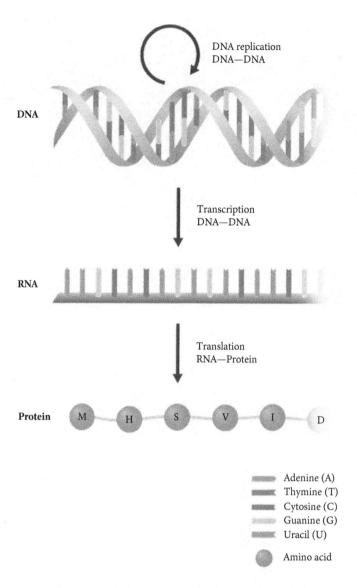

**Figure 9.6.** Further detailed illustration of the "central dogma" of molecular biology. The blocks connecting the two strands of the DNA double helix represent hydrogen bonds between the nitrogenous bases adenine (A) with thymine (T) and guanine (G) with cytosine (C). The nature and genetic coding significance of the pairings was the remarkable result of the birth of molecular biology as described in Chapter 6. Reproduced from National Human Genome Research Institute, genome.gov

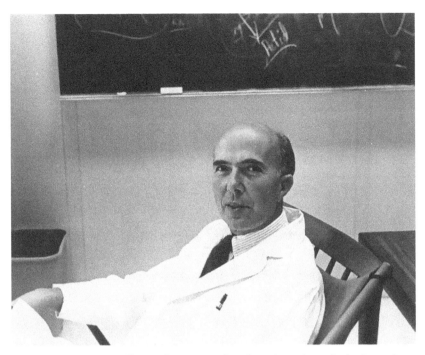

**Figure 9.7.** Renato Dulbecco (1914–2012). Italian-American virologist and geneticist at Cal Tech and the Salk Institute in California, who discovered virus-based gene transfer as a basis for transforming effect and who thereby laid the groundwork for the development of gene transferring and potentially therapeutic viruses. He received the 1975 Nobel Prize in Physiology or Medicine. Reproduced from National Institutes of Health.

*Restriction enzymes.* Probably the most important technical development in the evolution of molecular biology was the discovery of restriction enzymes, the core component underlying recombinant DNA technology. The advent of recombinant DNA technology (which came to be known as "gene splicing") made it possible to isolate and purify specific genes, to alter them and to move them from one organism to another, possibly even into human beings with the obvious long-term potential of manipulating human genetics, human disease and human evolution. The landmark studies that led to this remarkable new technology in biology came beginning in 1968 from the discovery, by the Swiss biochemist Werner Arber (Figure 9.11) and in the early 1970s by the groups of Matthew Meselson at Harvard University, Hamilton Smith and Daniel Nathans at Johns Hopkins University, of

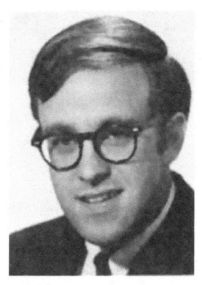

**Figure 9.8.** Richard Roblin. Reproduced with permission from R. Roblin.

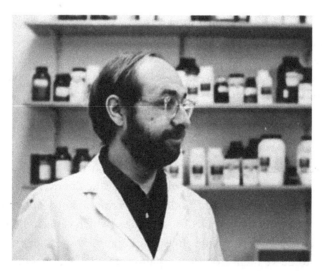

**Figure 9.9.** Theodore Friedmann (b. 1935). Viennese-American physician and geneticist who proposed the potential and the need for human gene therapy in 1972 with his colleague Richard Roblin following his studies with Frederick Sanger, Christian Anfinsen, J. Edwin Seegmiller, John Subak-Sharpe and Renato Dulbecco. He received the Japan Prize in 2015.

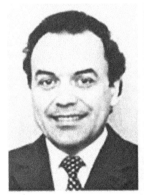

Figure 9.10. Science publication in 1972 by Theodore Friedmann and Richard Roblin describing the need for gene-based methods for therapy and the possibility for development of engineered viruses to introduce therapeutic genes into cells. The paper is considered a foundational publication in gene therapy. Reproduced from Tonse NK Raju, The Nobel Chronicles, *The Lancet*, 354/9189 (1999) with permission from Elsevier

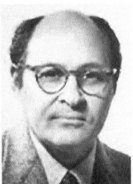
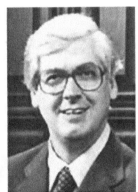

Figure 9.11. Werner Arber (b. 1929), Daniel Nathans (1928–1999) and Hamilton Smith (b. 1931). Geneticists and biochemists, these Swiss (Arber) and American scientists discovered the existence and function of bacteria-based restriction enzymes, core technologies for recombinant DNA science, for which they shared the 1978 Nobel Prize in Physiology or Medicine

"restriction" endonuclease enzymes that produce sequence-specific breaks in DNA and their applications to questions in molecular genetics.

The existence of these enzymes made possible the construction of hybrid recombinant DNA molecules consisting of genetic information from disparate organisms into one functional DNA molecule. In other words, the design of new organisms expressing new genetic functions.

Paul Berg (Figure 9.12), a biochemist at Stanford University, was studying gene expression in mammalian cells, and he was aware that Renato Dulbecco had just proven that the DNA tumor viruses SV40 and polyoma brought about tumorigenic changes in infected mammalian cells by introducing a transforming gene into the infected cell genome in a heritable and functional form. During a sabbatical year in the Dulbecco laboratory, Berg came to realize that viruses held the secret to how to transfer functional foreign genetic information into mammalian cells. Berg realized that these and probably other viruses could be used to create recombinant viruses as transducing agents to transfer foreign DNA into mammalian cells. In 1975, Berg reported that he successfully constructed a recombinant DNA molecule consisting of sequences from both the SV40 virus and the phage lambda.

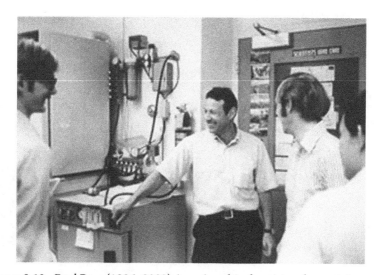

Figure 9.12. Paul Berg (1926–2023) American biochemist and geneticist who developed many of the concepts and techniques for recombinant DNA technology, including the construction of the first SV-40-based recombinant gene transfer vector. He shared the 1980 Nobel Prize in Chemistry with Frederick Sanger and Walter Gilbert. Courtesy of National Library of Medicine.

BIRTH OF MOLECULAR BIOLOGY AND RECOMBINANT DNA 77

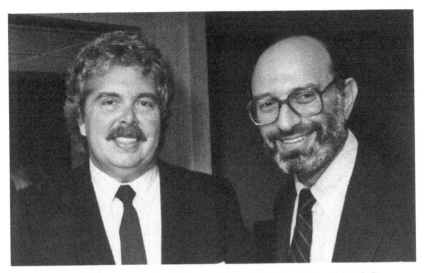

**Figure 9.13.** Herbert Boyer (left) (b. 1936) and Stanley Cohen (right) (b. 1935). As founder of the Biotech firm Genentech (Boyer) and professor of genetics at Stanford (Cohen), they developed, patented and commercialized the construction and use of recombinant DNA molecules. Courtesy of Stanley Cohen

This first construction of a recombinant DNA molecule set molecular genetics in general and the march toward human gene therapy into new and exciting directions. For their epochal work on the discovery and use of restriction enzymes, Arber, Smith and Nathans shared the 1978 Nobel Prize in Medicine or Physiology, and Berg shared the 1980 Nobel Prize in Chemistry with the discoverers of DNA sequencing technology Fred Sanger and Walter Gilbert.

At the same time and in the neighboring intellectual setting of Stanford University and the nearby University of California San Francisco, Hebert Boyer (b. 1936) and Stanley Cohen (b. 1935) for the first time constructed recombinant DNA molecules from disparate species such as *E. coli* and the clawed frog *Xenopus* (Figure 9.13).

***Reverse transcriptase.*** The explosive impact of the advent of recombinant DNA technology added go the revolutionary discovery by Howard Temin (Figure 9.14) and Satoshi Mizutani at the University of Wisconsin and David Baltimore at MIT of an enzyme in the virions of RNA viruses that to some observers seemed to challenge the central molecular biology dogma of the

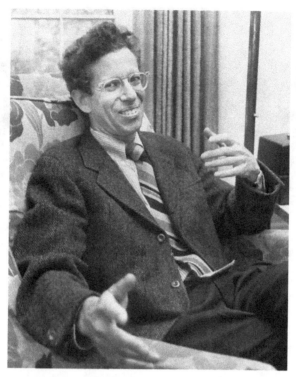

**Figure 9.14.** Howard Temin (1934–1994). American virologist and discoverer of reverse transcriptase. He shared the 1975 Nobel Prize in Physiology or Medicine with Renato Dulbecco and David Baltimore. Courtesy of Associated Press.

flow of genetic information from DNA to RNA to protein. While Temin was working with the well-known Rous sarcoma virus, he recognized that some of the infected cells displayed stable and heritable changes in infected cells. But since the Rous sarcoma virus had an RNA genome, how could an RNA virus bring about such permanent and heritable changes in the DNA genome of an infected cell? Temin concluded intuitively that that puzzle could best be explained by the existence of a double-stranded DNA intermediate form of the virus single-stranded RNA genome—a structure that he called the "provirus"—and that the virus must contain a function that carried out that change from RNA to DNA. As brilliantly correct as his intuition was, he and his studies were initially widely derided by the genetics and virology communities for seemingly daring, without rigorous proof, to undermine the "central dogma" of the flow of genetic information from DNA to RNA to protein.

At the same time, David Baltimore (Figure 9.15), working with the different RNA-based virus—the mouse leukemia virus (MLV)—independently identified an RNA-dependent DNA polymerase in virions of the virus. These epochal studies by Temin's and Baltimore's groups were published back-to-back in *Nature*, and the journal's cell biology correspondent John Tooze coined the term "reverse transcriptase" to underscore its apparent partial reversal of the flow of genetic information as pronounced by Crick's "central dogma." The discovery of the reverse transcriptase earned the name of "retroviruses" for the viruses studied by Temin and Baltimore and many other RNA genome viruses and earned them the 1975 Nobel Prize in Physiology or Medicine.

*DNA sequencing.* Understanding the structure of resulting recombinant DNAs and planning their construction was immensely facilitated by the development in the mid-1970s of methods to determine their nucleotide sequence. Principal among these methods were the chemical-based methods of Walter Gilbert (Figure 9.16) and Alan Maxam at Harvard University

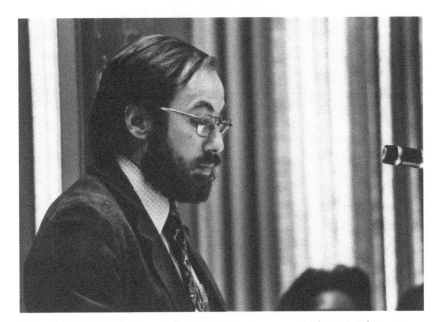

**Figure 9.15.** David Baltimore (b. 1938). Co-discoverer with Howard Temin of reverse transcriptase and co-winner with Temin and Dulbecco of the 1975 Nobel Prize in Physiology or Medicine. Courtesy of National Library of Medicine.

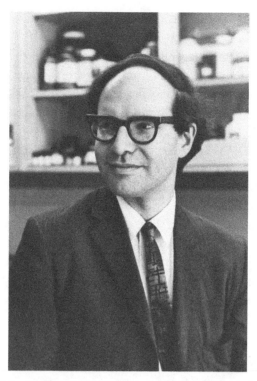

**Figure 9.16.** Walter Gilbert (b. 1932). American biochemist and molecular biologist, Gilbert with his Harvard colleague Allan Maxam developed the chemical-based technique for determining the sequence of bases in DNA. He shared the 1980 Nobel Prize in Chemistry with Frederick Sanger who had devised an alternative and more useful enzymic methodology for determining DNA sequence. Courtesy of Cold Spring Harbor Laboratory Archives.

and the enzymic methods developed by Fred Sanger at the Laboratory of Molecular Biology at Cambridge University. Although the chemical approach taken by Maxam and Gilbert was a major step forward (Figure 9.17), it was the methodology developed by Sanger that made a greater impact on most of the subsequent sequencing applications that have revolutionized nucleic acid sequencing and that now allow full sequence determination of entire mammalian genomes in hours to days rather than the 13 years required for the first complete sequencing of the human genome by the Human Genome Consortium from 1990 to 2003. The two remarkable sequencing technologies earned Paul Berg, Walter Gilbert and Fred Sanger the 1980

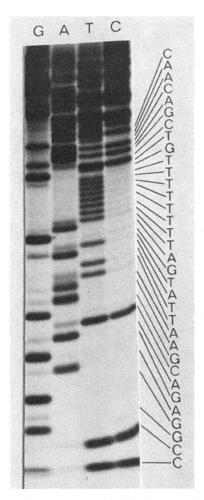

**Figure 9.17.** Thin layer electrophoresis by Theodore Friedmann of a portion of the genome of bacteriophage PhiX174 using the Gilbert-Maxam sequencing methods. The sequence is read upwards starting from the most rapidly moving fragments toward the bottom of the gel. Courtesy of T. Friedmann.

Nobel Prize in Chemistry, in Sanger's case, his second prize in that category (see Figure 9.18).

Using these revolutionary new techniques of gene "splicing" and reverse transcriptase, it suddenly became possible to isolate, purify ("clone") and characterize genes from any and all species, including humans. With relatively simple enzymatic steps, messenger RNA from cells could be converted in vitro into "complementary" DNA (cDNA) that then could be inserted by

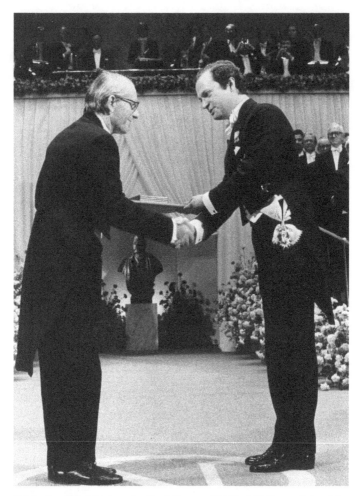

**Figure 9.18.** English biochemist Fred Sanger (1918–2013) receiving his second Nobel Prize in Chemistry (1980) from the king of Sweden. He is one of only five scientists who have ever received two Nobel prizes, including Marie Curie, Linus Pauling, John Bardeen and Barry Sharpless. Courtesy of TT/Sipa USA.

recombinant DNA methods into bacterial viral genomes, introduced into bacteria and thereby amplified and even made to produce large amounts of the encoded protein gene products. In 1979 Boyer, at the newly established biotech company refers to Genentech, and his colleagues Arthur Riggs and Keiichi Itakura, at the City of Hope Hospital in Duarte, California, used these powerful new recombinant DNA technologies to synthesize medically

BIRTH OF MOLECULAR BIOLOGY AND RECOMBINANT DNA 83

and commercially valuable proteins such as somatostatin (1) and of course insulin in genetically modified bacteria (2). Synthetic insulin became the first biological agent ever to be approved by the U.S. FDA. Shortly after these ground-breaking results, similar applications to the production of important gene-based pharmaceuticals came through the cloning of the genes for hemophilias A (3) and B (4) and their use for production of the clotting

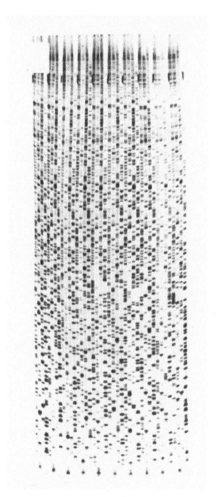

Figure 9.19. DNA sequencing gel with early generation of the Sanger dideoxy enzymatic sequencing technology, demonstrating increased efficiency compared with the Gilbert-Maxam technology. Courtesy of National Human Genome Research Institute, genome.gov

factors for millions of patients. Those results signaled the beginnings of the new and massively profitable era of genetic engineering and commercially valuable biotechnology (Figure 9.19).

### Reference

1. Itakura K, Hirose T, Crea R, Riggs AD, Heyneker HL, Bolivar F, Boyer HW. Expression in *Escherichia coli* of a chemically synthesized gene for the hormone somatostatin. *Science*. Dec 1977; Vol. 198(4321):1056–1063.

# 10

# Potential misstep becomes reality— the emergence of federal oversight and regulation

By 1980, major progress had been made in understanding the basis of many human diseases and, with the help of the recombinant DNA technology, even in isolating and characterizing the genes and aberrant genetic mechanisms responsible for disease. The underlying problem of transferring DNA into mammalian cells is the fact that the DNA molecule is negatively charged and therefore it cannot easily pass into or through the negatively charged mammalian cell membrane. Methods were required to neutralize or bypass this problem of electrical charge interference. Some of the most important resulting methods for circumventing this physical problem and for introducing foreign nucleic acids into mammalian cells (transfection) included electrical and chemically mediated techniques for efficiently introducing cloned nucleic acids into mammalian cells.

The earliest method of efficiently transfecting mammalian cells was with the use of diethylaminoethyl (DEAE)-dextran, a polycationic form of the carbohydrate polymer dextran that binds to the negatively charged backbone of nucleic acids and thus allows the foreign genetic material to enter cells by endocytosis. The method was first used by Joseph Pagano and Antti Vaheri in 1965 to facilitate plaque assays of poliovirus RNA in tissue cultures cells. With the exception of direct DEAE-dextran plasmid delivery in tumor gene therapy studies, the toxicity of DEAE has prevented its more widespread in vivo use in gene therapy studies.

In 1982, the German cell biologist Eberhard Neumann and his colleagues demonstrated that exposure of mouse cell suspensions to short high voltage electrical pulses allowed the enhanced entry of plasmids expressing the herpes thymidine kinase (TK) gene and the resulting stable expression of the foreign TK gene. This method of "electroporation" was found in many later studies to be an efficient method of making cell membranes permeable

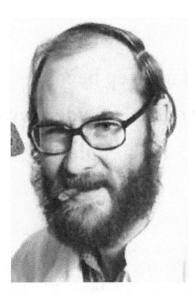

**Figure 10.1a.** Frank Graham, Canadian virologist. Together with his Dutch mentor and colleague Alex van der Eb, Dr. Graham developed the highly useful calcium phosphate method for introducing foreign DNA into eukaryotic cells. The technology became a gold standard for nonviral genetic modification of mammalian cells and is in wide use to the present day.

to foreign nucleic acids and drugs but, unsurprisingly, to be harsh and even harmful to cells. It has been adapted for use in vivo for gene transfer into a variety of tissues, especially muscle. Advantage has been taken of the toxicity of the technique in the form of stronger electrical pulses to create "irreversible" electroporation intended to cause cell death that has received interest for a variety of cancers, including prostate cancer, pancreatic cancer, melanoma and others. Outside of irreversible electroporation for cancer, in vivo electroporation has received very limited use in human gene therapy studies (1).

In 1973, the Canadian virologist Frank Graham (Figure 10.1a) and the Dutch virologist Alexander Van der Eb (b. 1934) (Figure 10.1b) discovered that they could vastly enhance the infectivity of adenovirus DNA by adding calcium phosphate to the transfection procedure. Calcium phosphate transfection represents a major turning point in molecular genetics and remains today one of the most efficient and widely used methods for introducing foreign DNA into mammalian and other eukaryotic cells.

Graham then followed up in 1977 with the demonstration that the calcium phosphate method allowed the efficient transfer of the herpes simplex

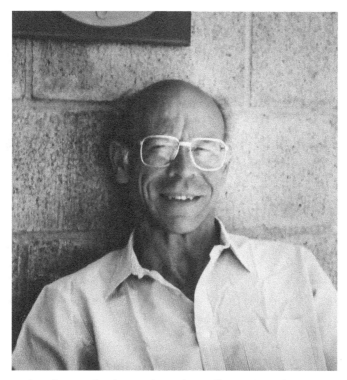

**Figure 10.1b.** Alex van de Eb, Dutch virologist (b. 1934). Molecular virologist who developed the useful calcium phosphate method for genetically modifying (transfecting) mammalian and other eukaryotic cells with foreign DNA.

thymidine kinase (TK) gene into human TK-deficient cells (2), and Michael Wigler and his team at Columbia University used the same transfection method to demonstrate similarly efficient transfer of the gene encoding adenosine phosphribosyltransferase (aprt) into murine aprt-deficient cells (3).

Bolstered by these powerful new demonstrations of efficient transfection into mammalian cells and by the availability of cloned and purified human disease-related genes, the stage was set for the first attempt at clinical gene therapy. One of the most tempting disease models for this revolutionary and daring work was the common and devastating genetic disease beta-thalassemia, a defect of production of the beta chain of hemoglobin leading to the life-threatening defect in blood production. One of the most likely biomedical centers for this work to be carried out was the laboratory of Martin Cline, a professor of medicine at UCLA in Los Angeles and a highly respected clinical hematologist and molecular biologist (Figure 10.2).

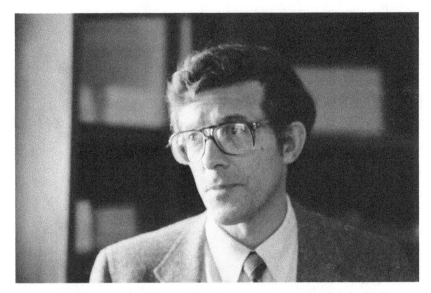

Figure 10.2. Martin Cline (b. 1934), American physician, molecular biologist and gene therapy investigator at the University of California Los Angeles. Courtesy of Martin Cline.

In 1980, Cline designed a gene therapy trial that involved isolation of bone marrow cells from patients with beta-thalassemia, genetically correcting them by calcium phosphate transfection with a cloned recombinant beta-globin gene followed by transfusion of the presumably genetically corrected cells into the patients' circulation (4). It was expected that the genetically corrected cells would find their way to a site in the bone marrow of the leg that had been made receptive for new cells by local irradiation. Cline's team had carried out model studies in the mouse that they interpreted to show that cells genetically modified to express different foreign genes could indeed be successfully transfused into mice and could express new genetic information in the animals.

Encouraged by his preliminary published mouse studies and additional experiments, some of which remained unpublished at the time, in 1980, Cline and colleagues used the available cloned hemoglobin beta chain cDNA (complementary DNA) and the calcium phosphate gene transfection method to design a gene therapy trial aimed at the genetic correction of defective globin gene expression by transforming bone marrow cells from two beta-thalassemia patients. After exposure in vitro of the patient's defective bone marrow cells and what he presumed would be genetic correction of the genetic defect in the cells, Cline transfused the presumably genetically modified cells back into the patients' circulation, hoping that they would not only express beta globin but also find their way to a portion of the leg bone marrow that he had irradiated to prepare a site for the genetically modified cells to allow them go become permanent residents in the bone marrow, to produce the newly introduced beta globin gene and thereby to correct the disease.

As he was required to do as a faculty member at UCLA, Cline submitted his proposed human trial to the UCLA Institutional Review Board for formal institutional approval. Unfortunately, after many months delay, the committee failed to approve the study and finally disapproved it. Cline, even without UCLA approval responded by arranging to carry out the study on two beta-thalassemia patients in Italy and Israel. He indeed had received approval from the human subjects review committee in Israel, but unfortunately their approval was not given for the precise recombinant DNA study that Cline carried out. In contrast, Cline had not received approval from the Italian authorities.

The decision by Cline to proceed with the clinical trial in 1980 was disastrous for him and for the nascent field of gene therapy (5). He was required to obtain permission from his home university for any clinical study carried out anywhere in the world, but he failed to do so. The experiment received very widespread attention in the medical, genetic and general public communities, most of which was harshly critical of the experimental design, citing the almost assured likelihood that the study would fail because of the lack of carefully controlled preliminary studies of long-term survival and foreign gene expression that would be necessary for the experiment to be successful. These studies constituted not only a major calamity for Dr. Cline but also a severe setback for the embryonic field of gene therapy. There was widespread scientific, medical and public condemnation of the field of gene therapy just as it was trying to gain a foothold as a legitimate new field of medicine.

To make matters worse for Cline, he lost his well-earned high clinical reputation at UCLA, had his National Institutes of Health (NIH) grants terminated and lost his faculty position at the university. Follow-up studies on the treated patients failed to show long-term survival of the transfused cells, adequate expression of the transfected beta-globin gene or any detectable clinical improvement. It was a very inauspicious start to this fledgling field.

## References

1. Neumann E, Schaefer-Ridder M, Wang Y, Hofschneider PH. Gene transfer into mouse lyoma cells by electroporation in high electric fields. *EMBO J.* 1982;1(7):841–845. doi: 10.1002/j.1460-2075.1982.tb01257.x.
2. Bacchetti S, Graham FL. Transfer of the gene for thymidine kinase to thymidine kinase-deficient human cells by purified herpes simplex viral DNA. *Proc Natl Acad Sci U S A.* 1977 Apr;74(4):1590–1594. doi: 10.1073/pnas.74.4.1590.
3. Wigler M, Pellicer A, Silverstein S, Axel R, Urlaub G, Chasin L. DNA-mediated transfer of the adenine phosphoribosyltransferase locus into mammalian cells. *Proc Natl Acad Sci U S A.* 1979 Mar;76(3):1373–1376. doi: 10.1073/pnas.76.3.1373.
4. Cline MJ. Perspectives for gene therapy: inserting new genetic information into mammalian cells by physical techniques and viral vectors. *Pharm. Ther.* 1985;29:69–92.
5. Kolata GB, Wade N. Human gene treatment stirs new debate. *Science.* 1980 Oct;210(4468):407. doi: 10.1126/science.6933693.

## Further reading

1. Committee on the Independent Review and Assessment of the Activities of the NIH Recombinant DNA Advisory Committee; Board on Health Sciences Policy; Institute of Medicine; Lenzi RN, Altevogt BM, Gostin LO, editors. *Oversight and Review of Clinical Gene Transfer Protocols: Assessing the Role of the Recombinant DNA Advisory Committee.* Washington, DC: National Academies Press (US); 2014 Mar 27. 3, Oversight of Gene Transfer Research. Available from: https://www.ncbi.nlm.nih.gov/books/NBK195894/.
2. Committee on the Independent Review and Assessment of the Activities of the NIH Recombinant DNA Advisory Committee; Board on Health Sciences Policy; Institute of Medicine; Lenzi RN, Altevogt BM, Gostin LO, editors. *Oversight and Review of Clinical Gene Transfer Protocols: Assessing the Role of the Recombinant DNA Advisory Committee.* Washington, DC: National Academies Press (US); 2014 Mar 27. 1, Introduction. Available from: https://www.ncbi.nlm.nih.gov/books/NBK195890/.
3. Wivel NA. Historical perspectives pertaining to the NIH Recombinant DNA Advisory Committee. *Human Gene Therapy.* 2014;25:19–24.

# 11

# Oversight and regulation of recombinant DNA research—the Asilomar conferences

The many remarkable new genetic techniques created over the previous several decades produced a new kind of genetics science that was no longer merely descriptive. Rather, it had become a manipulative science that permitted new ways to produce agents to treat human disease and has made virtually all human traits in health or in disease potential targets for genetic modification, for good, for ill or for mere whimsy. By the 1960s, this manipulative potential for genetics in medicine was beginning to be recognized by an increasing number of geneticists and other scientists. In 1966, Joshua Lederberg (1925–2008), together with his colleague Norton Zinder, showed that bacteriophages can transfer new genes into host organisms by a process that they called "genetic transduction." Lederberg predicted and supported the potential use of genetic manipulation to correct human disease, but also became alarmed about potential application of such new genetic power to pursue what he saw to be the harmful goals of the early English and American eugenic movements.

Similarly, the geneticist Robert Sinsheimer (1920–2017) saw the potential beneficial applications of molecular biology and virus-mediated gene transfer to understand and even treat human disease, but expressed deep scientific and ethical concern about the ability to use the astounding new tools of molecular biology and genetics to design and modify human biology and evolution before the potential benefits and dangers of such manipulations are fully understood.

*The Asilomar conferences.* In addition to the emerging ethical concerns about potential human genetic manipulation, there were extremely troubling concerns about the safety of some kinds of molecular biological research, especially those studies involving insertion of tumor virus genetic information into microorganisms such as *E. coli* that inhabit the human gastrointestinal system. Beginning in 1973, those concerns led Paul Berg and colleagues to organize a series of meetings at MIT, at the Asilomar Conference Center in

Pacific Grove, California, and at the Gordon Conference on Nucleic Acids to discuss potential hazards, particularly to scientists themselves, of some kinds of recombinant DNA experiments involving viruses. Interestingly, concerns about recombinant DNA research and the potential for environmental release of such molecules were not included in that first Asilomar meeting or in its final summary report. The obvious and glaring need for a much broader study of potential biohazards of recombinant DNA research, how they might be contained and the possible need for a moratorium on some kinds of studies led Berg and Maxine Singer (Figure 11.1) and their colleagues to organize a second conference at Asilomar in 1975, focused on the safety issues for human health and for the environment surrounding recombinant DNA studies. The meeting established principles defining the choice of appropriate disabled bacteria as host cells and the required use of disabled bacteria unable to survive outside the lab. The conference recommended that some kinds of experiments such as those involving known carcinogens or toxins and creating highly pathogenic organisms be forbidden.

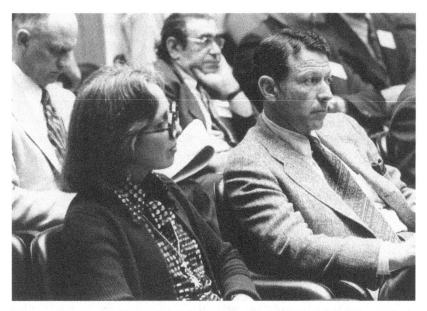

**Figure 11.1.** Maxine Singer (American molecular biologist, b. 1931) and Paul Berg at the 1976 NIH Director's meeting on recombinant DNA research. Reproduced from The Paul Berg Papers, *Profiles in Science*, National Library of Medicine.

This second Asilomar conference thereby established a strong social conscience for recombinant DNA research, one that emphasized the principle of self-regulation in science and a voluntary moratorium for this new and controversial field of science.

Deeply sensitive to the growing concerns of the genetics community, the National Institutes of Health (NIH) Director Donald Frederickson (Figure 11.2) created NIH Recombinant DNA Advisory Committee (RAC) that set about creating the *NIH Guidelines for Research Involving Recombinant DNA Molecules* that was then codified into official NIH policy when it was published in June 1976 in the *Federal Register*. The guidelines set standard procedures for research in this area and set out the need to oversee federally funded research with recombinant DNA technology. The guidelines quickly became the international model for oversight and, in the United States, set the operational standards for NIH review and approval of federally funded

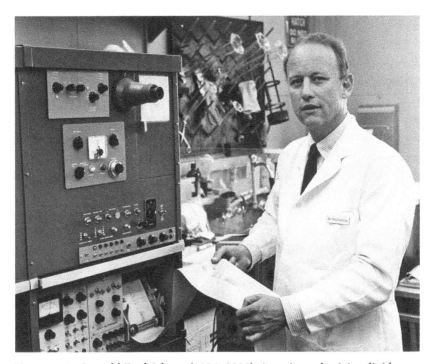

**Figure 11.2.** Donald Fredrickson (1924–2002), American physician, lipid metabolism pioneer and director of the U.S. National Institutes of Health 1975–1981. The Donald S. Fredrickson Papers, *Profiles in Science*, The National Library of Medicine.

grant support for recombinant DNA research. Because the committee consisted largely of bacterial geneticists, its expertise was targeted mostly at the safety of the recombinant DNA techniques per se and not, at that early stage, at human gene therapy applications.

It is important to recognize that the Asilomar conferences did not discuss in detail or make recommendations regarding most of the public policy and ethical concerns of recombinant DNA technology. In response to a growing and widespread concern throughout the genetic community about the ethical and policy uncertainties of recombinant DNA technology, the scientific and biomedical communities took several important steps to understand and to resolve these ethical and scientific fears. In 1975, the NIH established the Recombinant DNA Advisory Committee (RAC) to "to provide recommendations to the NIH Director and a public forum for discussion of the scientific, safety, and ethical issues related to basic and clinical research involving recombinant or synthetic nucleic acid molecules." The RAC became the central governmental NIH-based function for evaluating and implementing all proposals dealing with gene therapy. It is important to realize that the Asilomar conferences did not discuss in detail or make recommendations regarding most of the public policy and ethical concerns of recombinant DNA technology.*

In the aftermath of the Asilomar meetings and in response to a growing and widespread concern and loss of confidence throughout the genetic community and the general public anxiety about the ethical and policy uncertainties of the potential for human "genetic engineering," the scientific and biomedical communities took several important steps to understand and to resolve these ethical and scientific fears.

In 1975, the U.S. government under the leadership of the NIH Director Donald Fredrickson established the Recombinant DNA Advisory Committee (RAC) "to provide recommendations to the NIH Director and a public forum for discussion of the scientific, safety, and ethical issues related to basic and clinical research involving recombinant or synthetic nucleic acid molecules (1,2)."

---

* For a detailed history of the Asilomar meetings, see D. Fredrickson, *Asilomar and Recombinant DNA: The End of the Beginning*, ed. Hanna KE (Washington, DC: National Academies Press (US), 1991). https://www.ncbi.nlm.nih.gov/books/NBK234217/.

The RAC promptly set about establishing the *NIH Guidelines for Research Involving Recombinant DNA Molecules* that were codified into formal NIH policy by publication in the Federal Register in 1976.

The RAC became the central governmental NIH-based agency for evaluating and implementing all proposals dealing with gene therapy.

Because of continuing scientific and public unease about what was coming to be called "genetic engineering" and objections from some conservative religious communities to humans "interfering with Nature" and proclaiming the need to respect the dignity of individual human beings, the government in 1982 established the *President's Commission for the Study of Ethical Problems in Medicine and Biomedical and Behavioral Research* that promptly produced the influential document *Splicing Life* that made a number of important recommendations on how to proceed safely and ethically with human genetic modification. Their document eased some of the concern in the scientific and public minds and greatly facilitated the extension of recombinant DNA technology to human gene therapy application.

The commission concluded that recombinant DNA technology posed no new ethical dilemmas or problems and that the RAC committee should include "public" and nonscientific members to increase its expertise in social and ethical issues. Furthermore, it was obvious that there needed to be more committee membership strength in matters more immediately concerned with potential human application, an awareness that led in 1983 to the establishment of the RAC Human Gene Therapy Subcommittee (HGTS) that in 1985 created a set of criteria, called the *Points to Consider in the Design and Submission of Somatic Cell Human Gene Therapy Protocols* for how to proceed with human studies. The "Points to Consider" were published in the *Federal Register* in 1985 and became codified as official NIH policy. They became a kind of road map for investigators who wished to develop gene therapy studies and rapidly became a "checklist" of components of gene therapy studies that would be required for acceptable applications for federal grant applications and for permission to proceed with their studies.

By 1988, the HGTS had compiled an exhaustive set of the kinds of clinical data that might be required for a human gene therapy trial in a document entitled *Preclinical Data Document* and very quickly received a proposal from W.F. Anderson, Steven Rosenberg and their colleagues at the NIH for a first human gene therapy trial. The door to human clinical gene therapy had been opened (3) (Figures 11.3 and 11.4).

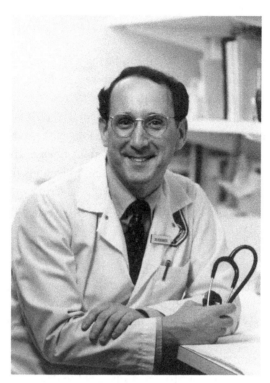

**Figure 11.3.** Steven Rosenberg (b. 1940), American physician, oncologist, molecular biologist and gene therapy investigator. Courtesy of National Cancer Institute ccr.cancer.gov/steven-a-rosenberg

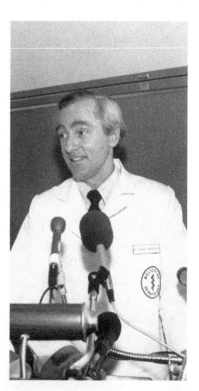

**Figure 11.4.** W. French Anderson (b. 1936), American physician, molecular biologist, gene therapy investigator. Courtesy of National Cancer Institute.

## References

1. Committee on the Independent Review and Assessment of the Activities of the NIH Recombinant DNA Advisory Committee; Board on Health Sciences Policy; Institute of Medicine; Lenzi RN, Altevogt BM, Gostin LO, editors. *Oversight and Review of Clinical Gene Transfer Protocols: Assessing the Role of the Recombinant DNA Advisory Committee.* Washington, DC: National Academies Press (US); 2014 Mar 27. 3, Oversight of Gene Transfer Research. Available from: https://www.ncbi.nlm.nih.gov/books/NBK195894/.
2. Committee on the Independent Review and Assessment of the Activities of the NIH Recombinant DNA Advisory Committee; Board on Health Sciences Policy; Institute of Medicine; Lenzi RN, Altevogt BM, Gostin LO, editors. *Oversight and Review of Clinical Gene Transfer Protocols: Assessing the Role of the Recombinant DNA Advisory Committee.* Washington, DC: National Academies Press (US); 2014 Mar 27. 1, Introduction. Available from: https://www.ncbi.nlm.nih.gov/books/NBK195890/.
3. Wivel, NA. Historical perspectives pertaining to the NIH Recombinant DNA Advisory Committee. *Human Gene Therapy.* 2014;25:19–24.

# 12
# Chemical nonviral vectors

For this new direction of human genetics to become a legitimate new force in medicine, major advances were required in two additional areas—the development of tools to isolate and purify disease-related genes, and the development of tools for introducing foreign and potentially therapeutic genetic information into human and other eukaryotic cells (i.e., gene transfer "vectors").

The first of these two needs was fulfilled in the 1970s through the advent of recombinant DNA technology as reviewed in earlier chapters. Geneticists were finally able to identify and localize the genes responsible for human disease and even to isolate them in large amounts in purified form. At approximately the same time, methods were becoming available to move genetic material into genetically marked eukaryotic cells to study gene regulation and in ways that might even allow correction of disease-causing mechanisms.

A number of chemical methods had been developed for transferring genetic material into mammalian cells, including DNA transfer mediated by DEAE-dextran and calcium phosphate. These positively charged agents facilitated the uptake of negatively charged nucleic acids through the negatively charged mammalian cell membranes and thereby made possible many in vitro tissue culture studies in mammalian cells. A variety of methods emerged that complemented the calcium phosphate, DEAE-dextran chemical-based procedures for delivering DNA into eukaryotic cells in vitro or even in vivo. Most notable among these methods was the synthetic cationic lipid approach pioneered by Philip Felgner (Figure 12.1) and colleagues at Syntex Corp. in Palo Alto and later at Vical Inc., a new start-up biotech company established in La Jolla, California. In 1987, Felgner developed N-[1-(2,3-dioleyloxy)propyl]-N,N,N-trimethylammonium chloride (DOTMA) (lipofectin) which became and remains to the present day one of the most widely used and important nonviral methods for introducing nucleic acids into mammalian cells (1).

The development of cationic lipid reagents for transfer and expression of foreign genetic information into eucaryotic cells facilitated many kinds of

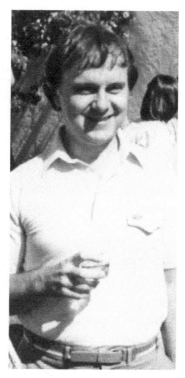

**Figure 12.1.** Phillip Felgner (b. 1950), American biochemist, molecular biologist and inventor of lipofection technology used in many aspects of molecular genetics research and recently most importantly in anti-COVID and other vaccines.

studies in mammalian and other eukaryotic cells, not only for delivery into mammalian cells of DNA transgenes but of RNA as well, as indicated by its central role in the development of mRNA-based vaccines during the global COVID pandemic that devastated much of the world beginning in 2020. Despite being declared formally over in 2023, COVID continues in endemic form to this day and is likely to remain so. The striking success by the pharmaceutical and biotech companies Pfizer and Moderna in creating highly effective vaccines for COVID-19 was based on the use of liposome-based vectors for mRNA transfer and the striking work of Drew Weissman and Katalin Kariko at the University of Pennsylvania (Figure 12.2). That remarkable scientific achievement relied on use of the nucleoside-modified mRNA-encoding viral antigens (replacement of uridine with pseudouridine in the mRNA to reduce the immunogenicity of mRNA) combined with efficient

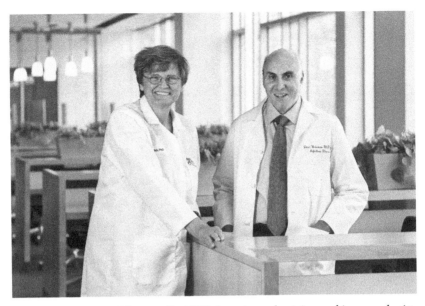

**Figure 12.2.** Drew Weissman (b. 1959) American physician and immunologist, and Hungarian biochemist Katalin Kariko (b. 1955), who established the scientific technologies for the development of mRNA vaccines, such as those used in the prevention of infection with COVID-19 virus.

delivery by lipid nanoparticles. Those changes have become a platform for effective delivery of mRNA not only for vaccine development but possibly even for revolutionizing much wider gene therapy applications, including cancer (2).

Simultaneous with the development of this lipofection technique came additional advances in the chemistry of nucleic acid–polymer interactions and in nonviral gene transfer techniques that resulted in the development by Ernst Wagner (Figure 12.3) and Matt Cotten (Figure 12.4) in Vienna and many other geneticists and cell biologists of additional polycation formulations for nucleic acid delivery (3). While these techniques have facilitated many further studies of cell biology and gene transfer, their usefulness for widespread clinically relevant applications has yet in most cases to be established.

In a surprising development, during the same time Jon Wolff (Figure 12.5) in Madison, Wisconsin, in collaboration with Felgner at Vical Inc. in La Jolla, found that it was possible to introduce and stably express foreign DNA in the form of naked plasmid DNA directly in vivo (4). The efficiency

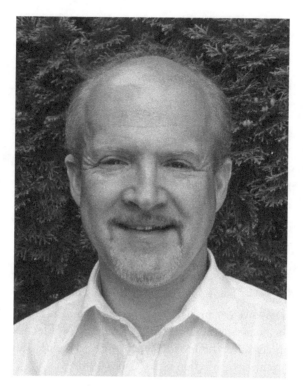

**Figure 12.3.** Ernst Wagner (b. 1960) German-Austrian virologist and development of nonviral techniques for gene transfer. Courtesy of Ernst Wagner.

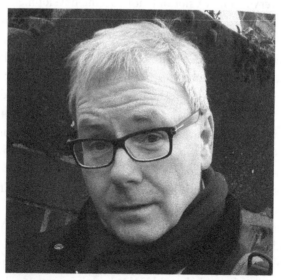

**Figure 12.4.** Matthew Cotton, (b. 1957) American virologist and developer of methods for genetic characterization of viral evolution.

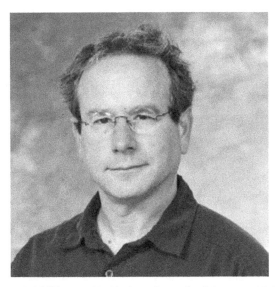

**Figure 12.5.** Jon Wolff (1956–2020). American physician, geneticist and molecular biologist who was the first to demonstrate introduction of foreign genetic material in the form of plasmids directly into muscle. Courtesy of Matthew Cotten.

of gene transfer by this method is generally low, and clinical utilization of naked nucleic acid gene transfer would require major technological improvement. Rapid large-volume injections of DNA plasmids and even RNA into the vasculature ("hydrodynamic" delivery) has improved gene transfer and lead to broad tissue distribution of transgene expression in rodents, particularly in tissues such as skeletal muscle and liver. But hydrodynamic delivery has not yet shown comparable efficacy in larger animals or in human clinical settings. Overall, except for their use for vaccine development, chemically mediated DNA or RNA delivery has until now not matured as quickly for therapeutic purposes as has the use of the biological agents—viruses—more suited to the task of nuclei acid transfer into eukaryotic cells.

### References

1. Felgner PL, Gadek TR, Holm M, Roman R, Chan HW, Wenz M, Northrop JP, Ringold GM, Danielsen M. Lipofection: a highly efficient, lipid-mediated DNA-transfection procedure. *Proc Natl Acad Sci U S A.* 1987 Nov;84(21):7413–7417. doi: 10.1073/pnas.84.21.7413.

2. Kariko K. Developing mRNA for therapy. *J Med.* 2022;71(1):31. doi: 10.2302/kjm.71-001-ABST. PMID: 35342149.
3. Zhang P, Wagner, E. History of polymeric gene delivery systems. *Top Curr Chem (Cham).* 2017 Apr;375(2):26. doi: 10.1007/s41061-017-0112-0. Epub 2017 Feb 8.PMID: 28181193 Review.
4. Wolff JA, Malone RW, Williams P, Chong W, Acsadi G, Jani A, Felgner PL. Direct gene transfer into mouse muscle in vivo. *Science.* 1990 Mar 23;247(4949 Pt 1):1465–1468. doi: 10.1126/science.1690918.

# 13

# Genetics—from a descriptive to a manipulative science

One solution to the problem of inefficient gene transfer with chemical and naked DNA or RNA methods lay in the use of the agents that existed in nature and that had evolved to do precisely that job (e.g., viruses). The theoretical basis for the use of viruses as agents for gene transfer had been foreseen in the 1960s and 1970s by geneticists such as Joshua Lederberg, Robert Sinsheimer, in the early studies of Stanfield Rogers, implied by the papova virus studies of Dulbecco and in the recombinant DNA studies by Berg.

In 1972, just before the advent of recombinant DNA technology, two postdoctoral fellows in the Dulbecco laboratory, Richard Roblin and I, proposed ways in which the remarkable new tools of molecular genetics could be used not merely to understand human genetic disease but in fact to develop new forms of treatment to correct the underlying genetic defect in those illnesses, especially using engineered viruses to carry the therapeutic DNA into diseased human cells (see Figure 9.10). The Friedmann–Roblin 1972 paper was conceptually based on the 1968 demonstration by Friedmann and his NIH colleagues Drs. Jay Seemiller and John Subak Sharpe that exposure of cultured fibroblasts from a patient with hypoxanthine-guanine phosphoribosyltransferase (HPRT)-deficiency Lesch–Nyhan disease to total cell DNA from HPRT-positive cells led to the appearance of HPRT enzymic activity in a very small number of exposed cells. The efficiency of the transformation event was exceedingly low, suggesting that a possible therapeutic application of this phenomenon would require the use of far more efficient methods for introducing foreign DNA into mammalian cells. At approximately the same time Renato Dulbecco and his Salk Institute colleagues demonstrated that papova viruses such as polyoma and SV40 cause tumorigenic changes in cells by stably introducing a portion of their genome encoding a tumor antigen (T) into infected mammalian cells. That publication (see Figure 9.10) was the first major publication to outline the opportunity and the need for virus-based gene transfer methods for gene therapy for human disease. It has been described as foundational for human gene therapy (2) and was cited by the award to Theodore Friedmann and Alain Fischer of the 2015 Japan Prize for the development of the concept and first clinical proof of principle for gene therapy (see Figure 13.1).

As oversight and regulatory apparatuses were being developed in the aftermath of the Asilomar meetings to establish safe and ethical applications of recombinant DNA technology, advances were being made in the design and use of genetically modified viruses to serve as efficient and safe delivery vehicles or "vectors" to introduce foreign DNA into mammalian and even human cells. A variety of viruses were candidates for such applications, including the early candidates such as Shope papilloma virus and the papova viruses.

*Papovaviruses—SV40 and polyoma.* Despite the early work by Paul Berg on a recombinant SV40-based virus vector, the transition to potential clinical

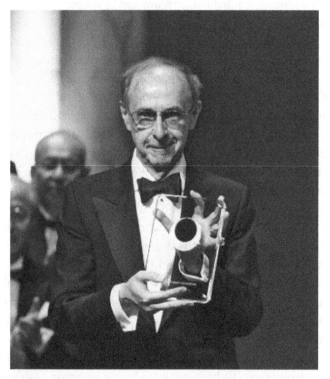

**Figure 13.1.** Theodore Friedmann receiving the 2015 Japan Prize for the development of gene therapy. He shared the prize with Alain Fischer of the Necker Hospital in Paris for his development of gene therapy for severe combined immunodeficiency Disease (SCID).

application was a much more difficult task and found little footing in the context of gene therapy. In 1979, his laboratory reported the synthesis of rabbit beta globin protein from a recombinant SV40 virus in cultured kidney cells, suggesting a possible approach to genetic correction of hematological disease (3). Similarly, also in 1979, Dean Hamer and Philip Leder at the NIH reported the production of mouse beta globin from an SV40 recombinant virus (4). Despite these enticing results, the interest in papova virus vectors for potential disease-related applications faded as interest grew in the development of other and more promising classes of virus vectors.

*Adenovirus vectors.* As interest in those virus systems waned, greater emphasis came to be put on the DNA-based adenoviruses as attractive candidates for gene transfer vector application. As early as 1971, adenovirus-based vaccines came into widespread use in the U.S military, and there was a high level of experience and confidence in their safety and efficacy. Furthermore, studies with adenoviruses had already played a major role in much of eukaryotic gene expression, including the discovery of introns and RNA splicing.

For these reasons, adenoviruses were poised to be reasonable early candidates for use as gene transferring vectors for potential application for human gene therapy. Adenoviruses are double-stranded DNA viruses with very broad mammalian host ranges and, in the human, capable of producing mild, usually upper respiratory disease to very severe, life-threatening multi-organ disease. Adenoviruses were among the first to be engineered and adapted as gene transfer vectors (5, 6) and were found to have several important advantages, including their ease of production, their broad host range including post-mitotic cells such as neurons and hepatocytes, their ability to produce high levels of transgene expression, their property to remain episomal rather than integrated into the host cell genome and thereby potentially disrupting vital host gene functions. Complicating their use for gene therapy applications is the fact that they are highly immunogenic and can therefore induce unwanted and physiologically dangerous release of chemokines and cytokines from infected mammalian cells. Adenoviruses and adenovirus vectors have also been shown to induce brisk immune responses not only to their capsid proteins but also to the proposed therapeutic transgene payload. Attempts to eliminate the problem of vector immunogenicity have included construction of "gutless" helper-dependent derivatives depleted of all viral protein-coding sequences and retaining only necessary cis-acting elements such as origins of viral DNA replication and packaging sequences, but immunogenicity remains a major problem for adenovirus vectors. It was precisely this property of immunogenicity and cytokine release that led to the death of an 18-year-old patient, Jesse Gelsinger, in a gene therapy trial of an adenovirus vector encoding the ornithine transcarbamylase (OTC) gene in 1999 (Figure 13.2).

*Retrovirus and lentivirus vectors.* The most significant and most important breakthroughs in the design of gene transfer vectors for gene therapy occurred in the 1980s and 1990s with the development of highly efficient derivatives of

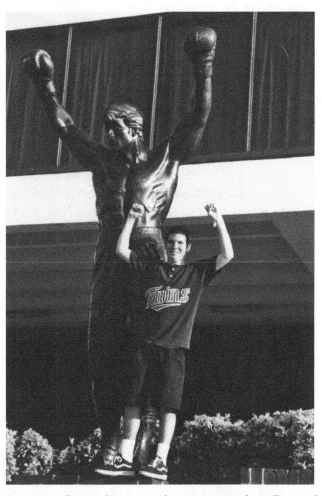

**Figure 13.2.** Jesse Gelsinger (1981–1999), posing as Rocky Balboa at the Philadelphia Museum of Art before his fatal participation in the University of Pennsylvania gene therapy trial for ornithine transcarbamylase. Courtesy of Dr. Paul Gelsinger.

several classes of RNA viruses, viruses that replicate by a process involving DNA copies of their RNA genomes and that integrate those DNA copies into infected cell genomes. They are members of the subfamily Orthoretroviridae and include alpha, beta, gamma, delta and epsilon retroviruses defined by the nature of their pathogenesis, the lentivirus subfamily such as the HIV virus and a subfamily of Spumaviruses. It was the Rous sarcoma and the mouse leukemia gamma retrovirus (MLV) that Temin and Baltimore used for their seminal discovery of reverse transcriptase. Members of the gamma retrovirus class, such as murine leukemia virus (MLV) were often preferred tools for both preclinical and even gene therapy clinical trial applications, but after 1996 they came to be supplanted by lentivirus.

In 1981 and 1982, laboratories led by Temin at the University of Wisconsin, David Baltimore at MIT, Edward Scolnick at the NIH (Figure 13.3) and Robert Weinberg at MIT (Figure 13.4) reported the construction

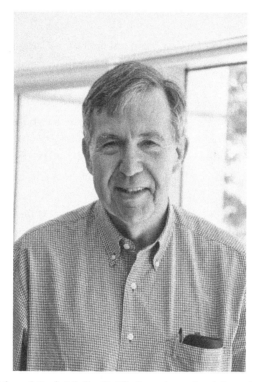

**Figure 13.3.** Edward Scolnick (b. 1941), American physician, virologist and molecular biologist at NIH, Harvard Medical School and Broad Institute, Cambridge, Massachusetts. Courtesy of Broad Institute/Dr. Scolnick.

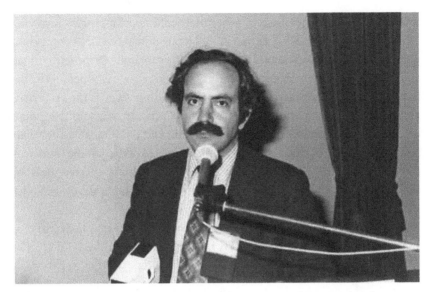

**Figure 13.4.** Robert Weinberg (b. 1942), American virologist, molecular biologist and cancer investigator at MIT. Courtesy of Robert Weinberg.

of retroviruses carrying foreign, nonviral genes (7–9), opening the door to construction of effective vectors expressing therapeutic genes.

The development of this powerful new technology for gene transfer, together with the enormous growth of human genetics added a sense of imminence to the concept of human gene therapy. These methods provided the tools for the first demonstration by Friedmann and his colleagues that a virally transferred transgene could correct genetic and biochemical elements of a disease phenotype, in this case HPRT-deficiency in Lesch–Nyhan disease (see Figure 13.5a) (10).

It also spurred the organization in 1983 of what was the first meeting devoted to the multiple dimensions of the emerging concept of gene therapy and brought together at the Banbury Center at the Cold Spring Harbor in New York many of the most influential leaders in the scientific, medical, ethical and legal communities to identify the opportunities and potential dangers inherent in the field of human gene therapy. The small meeting was summarized by Theodore Friedmann in the Banbury Center book *Gene Therapy: Fact and Fiction*, which introduced the field to the disparate biomedical and ethics communities (Figure 13.5b).

Many major technical advances over the 1990s brought the retrovirus vector transduction systems to a point where clinical application seemed more and more justifiable and even imminent. In 1991, the use of the capsid G protein of vesicular stomatitis virus for pseudotyping this class of viruses

# GENETICS—DESCRIPTIVE TO A MANIPULATIVE SCIENCE 111

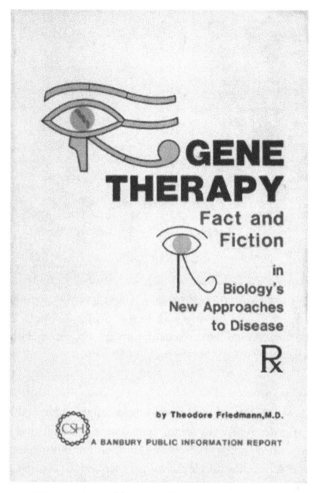

**Figure 13.5a.** 1982 meeting publication of the gene therapy symposium at the Banbury Center of the Cold Spring Harbor Laboratory in New York. The meeting was the first comprehensive multidisciplinary review of the nascent field of gene therapy that included participant molecular biologists, medical researchers and ethicists. Courtesy of Theodore Friedmann.

**Partial Phenotypic Correction of Human Lesch-Nyhan (Hypoxanthine-Guanine Phosphoribosyltransferase-deficient) Lymphoblasts with a Transmissible Retroviral Vector\***

(Received for publication, December 12, 1983)

Randall C. Willis[a], Douglas J. Jolly[b], A. Dusty Miller[c,d], Matthew M. Plent, Abby C. Esty, Paul J. Anderson, Hsiao-Chen Chang[e], Oliver W. Jones[e], J. Edwin Seegmiller[f], and Theodore Friedmann[b]

*From the Departments of Medicine and Pediatrics, University of California, San Diego, La Jolla, California 92093 and 'The Molecular Biology and Virology Laboratory, The Salk Institute, San Diego, California 92138*

**Figure 13.5b.** Report by Friedmann and colleagues of the partial phenotypic correction of the HPRT-deficiency disease phenotype in cultured lymphoblasts from a patient with Lesch-Nyhan Disease.

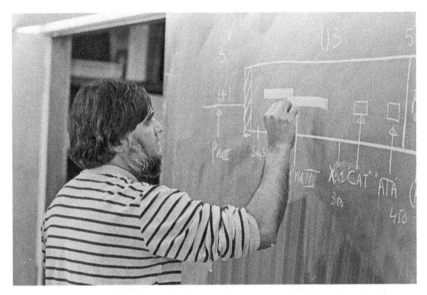

**Figure 13.6.** Inder Verma (b. 1947), Indian-American virologist, molecular biologist and gene therapy investigator from the Salk Institute in La Jolla, California during a symposium presentation at the Cold Spring Harbor Laboratory. Courtesy of Cold Spring Harbor Laboratory.

began to allow the production of broad host-range, stable and highly efficient gene transfer retrovirus vector preparations suitable and acceptable for human clinical application (10). Another groundbreaking advance occurred in 1996 with the development by Inder Verma (Figure 13.6), Didier Trono (Figure 13.7), Luigi Naldini (Figure 13.8) and their colleagues at the Salk Institute in La Jolla of vectors derived from the retrovirus subfamily of Lentiviruses that causes HIV (11, 12). These vectors provided important advantages over the gamma retrovirus vectors, including their ability to transduce terminally differentiated cells and, as came to be understood in later clinical studies, their more favorable and safer mechanisms of integration into host cell genomes resulting in their reduced potential for genotoxicity. For these reasons, the lentivirus vectors, especially those derived from the human HIV virus, have become one of the most effective and clinically favored gene transfer technologies.

*Adeno-associated virus vectors.* The Parvoviridiae family of adeno-associated viruses was discovered in 1965 by Robert Atchison and colleagues

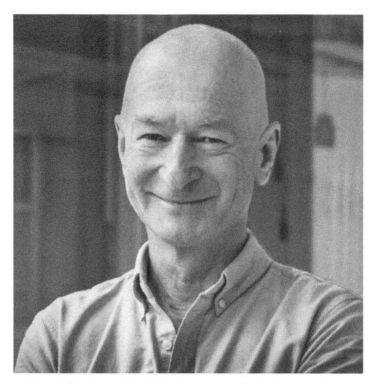

**Figure 13.7.** Didier Trono (b. 1956), Swiss molecular biologist and virologist. Currently professor at the Ecole Polytechnique Federale in Lausanne, Switzerland. Reproduced with kind permission from Professor Trono.

as a "contaminant" of adenovirus preparations. Adeno-associated viruses are small, non-enveloped single-stranded DNA viruses that require another "helper" virus such as adenovirus or herpes virus to replicate. Eleven naturally occurring adeno-associated virus (AAV) serotypes have been identified, with each serotype having distinct preferential tissue tropism. AAV viruses are largely nonpathogenic, although most humans are seropositive for one or another of the many serotypes even in the absence of known illness.

In 1984, Barrie Carter (Figure 13.9) at the U.S. National Institutes of Health and Nick Muzyczka (Figure 13.10) at the University of Florida took advantage of important previous cloning studies of AAV studies by Jude Samulski (Figure 13.11) of the University of Florida to construct the first gene transfer AAV vectors (13–15).

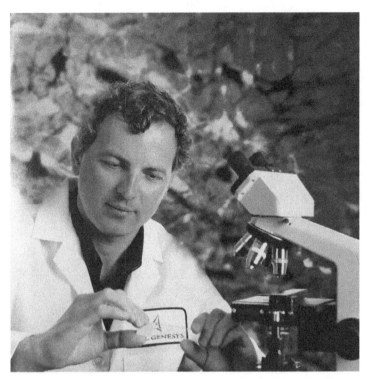

**Figure 13.8.** Luigi Naldini (b. 1959), Italian molecular and cell biologist, gene therapy investigator, during his work at the Salk Institute in La Jolla, California. Currently director of the Telethon Institute for Gene Therapy, Milan, Italy. Courtesy of Luigi Naldini.

In the past several years, the AAV viruses have become the most highly preferred virus platform for many human gene therapy applications. AAV vectors exist in an episomal state in the infected cell, and therefore, unlike the retrovirus and lentivirus vectors that integrate into host cell genomes, AAV vectors do not disrupt expression of host cell genes such as host cell oncogenes (genotoxicity). Additional advantages of AAV vectors include their ability to allow prolonged stable transgene expression from their episomal state in the cell, their much-reduced immunogenicity and their broad tissue tropism. AAV capsids have been highly engineered to create "pseudotyped" viruses that contain the genome of one serotype in the capsid of a different pseudotype, thereby permitting preferential and specific tissue-specific infection and gene delivery. In addition to standard pseudotypes,

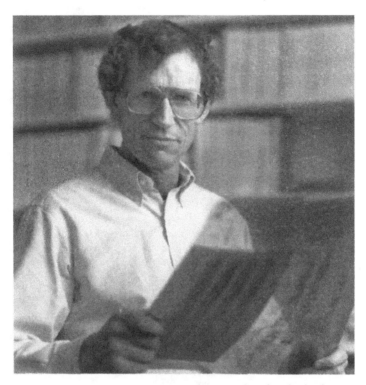

**Figure 13.9.** Barrie Carter, American Virologist and molecular biologist, gene therapy investigator shown during his time as laboratory chief at the National Institute of Diabetes and Digestive and Kidney Diseases at the U.S. National Institutes of Health. Courtesy of National Institutes of Health.

other AAV vectors have been created that contain capsids from several, even as many as eight, different AAV serotypes, a manipulation that can further alter the tissue tropism and increase targeting efficiency.

*Additional miscellaneous virus vectors.* In addition to adenoviruses, papova viruses, retro- and lentiviruses and adeno-associated viruses, attempts have been made to adapt a number of other viruses as gene transfer agents in mammalian and other eucaryotic systems, for both gene delivery and oncolytic purposes (13, 16, 17). These viruses have included recombinant enteroviruses such as coxsakie viruses, herpes viruses (18) and the foamy virus (FV) class of retroviruses. These therapy systems are largely at less well-developed stages and have not proven as useful or effective as the adenovirus, retro- and lentiviruses and adeno-associated viruses.

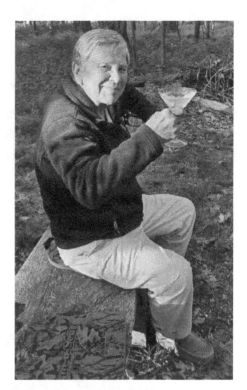

**Figure 13.10.** Nicholas Muzyczka (1947–2023), German-American virologist and a developer with his University of Florida colleagues Ken Berns, Jude Samulski and Terence Flotte of the AAV vector gene transfer technology.

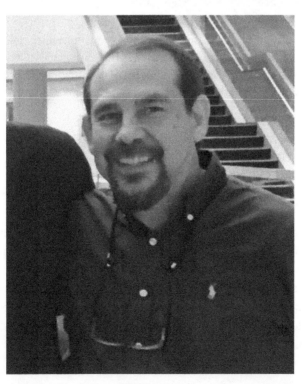

**Figure 13.11.** Richard Jude Samulski (b. 1954), American virologist and principal developer of the AAV vector gene transfer technology for gene therapy.

## References

1. Friedmann, T, Roblin, R. Gene therapy for human genetic disease? *Science.* 1972 Mar 3;175(4025):949–955. doi: 10.1126/science.175.4025.949.
2. Dunbar CE, High KA, Joung JK, Kohn DB, Ozawa K, Sadelain M. Gene therapy comes of age. *Science.* 2018 Jan 12;359(6372):eaan4672. doi: 10.1126/science.aan4672. PMID: 29326244 Review.
3. Mulligan RC, Howard BH, Berg P. Synthesis of rabbit beta-globin in cultured monkey kidney cells following infection with a SV40 beta-globin recombinant genome. *Nature.* 1979 Jan 11;277(5692):108–114. PubMed PMID: 215915.
4. Hamer DH, Leder P. Expression of the chromosomal mouse Beta maj-globin gene cloned in SV40. *Nature.* 1979 Sep 6;281(5726):35–40. PubMed PMID: 233122.
5. Haj-Ahmad Y, Graham FL. Development of a helper-independent human adenovirus vector and its use in the transfer of the herpes simplex virus thymidine kinase gene. *J Virol.* 1986 Jan;57(1):267–274.
6. Ballay A, Levrero M, Buendia MA, Tiollais P, Perricaudet M. In vitro and in vivo synthesis of the hepatitis B virus surface antigen and of the receptor for polymerized human serum albumin from recombinant human adenoviruses. *EMBO J.* 1985 Dec 30;4(13B):3861–3865. doi: 10.1002/j.1460 2075.1985.tb04158.x. PMID: 3004975.
7. Shimotohno K, Temin HM. Formation of infectious progeny virus after insertion of herpes simplex thymidine kinase gene into DNA of an avian retrovirus. *Cell.* 1981;26, 67–77.
8. Wei C, Gibson M, Spear PG, Scolnick EM. Construction and isolation of a transmissible retrovirus containing the src gene from Harvey murine sarcoma virus and the thymidine kinase gene from herpes simplex virus type 1. *J. Virol.* 1981;39, 935–944.
9. Tabin CJ, Hoffmann JW, Goff SP, Weinberg RA. Adaptation of a retrovirus as a eucaryotic vector transmitting the herpes simplex virus thymidine kinase gene. *Mol Cell Biol.* 1982 Apr;2(4):426–436. doi: 10.1128/mcb.2.4.426-436.1982.
10. Willis RC, Jolly DJ, Miller AD, Plent MM, Esty AC, Anderson PJ, Chang HC, Jones OW, Seegmiller JE, Friedmann T. Partial phenotypic correction of human Lesch-Nyhan (hypoxanthine-guanine phosphoribosyltransferase-deficient) lymphoblasts with a transmissible retroviral vector. *J Biol Chem.* 1984 Jun 25;259(12):7842–7849.
11. Emi N, Friedmann T, Yee JK. Pseudotype formation of murine leukemia virus with the G protein of vesicular stomatitis virus. *J Virol.* 1991 Mar;65(3):1202–1207. doi: 10.1128/JVI.65.3.1202-1207.1991.
12. Naldini L, Blömer U, Gallay P, Ory D, Mulligan R, Gage FH, Verma IM, Trono D. In vivo gene delivery and stable transduction of nondividing cells by a lentiviral vector. *Science.* 1996 Apr 12;272(5259):263–267. doi: 10.1126/science.272.5259.263.
13. Naldini L, Trono D, Verma IM. Lentiviral vectors, two decades later. *Science.* 2016 Sep 9;353(6304):1101–1102. doi: 10.1126/science.aah6192.
14. Hermonat PL, Labow MA, Wright R, Berns KI, Muzyczka N. Genetics of adeno-associated virus: isolation and preliminary characterization of adeno-associated virus type 2 mutants. *J Virol.* 1984 Aug;51(2):329–339. doi: 10.1128/JVI.51.2.329-339.1984. PMID: 6086948.
15. Tratschin JD, Miller IL, Carter BJ. Genetic analysis of adeno-associated virus: properties of deletion mutants constructed in vitro and evidence for an adeno-associated virus replication function. *J Virol.* 1984 Sep;51(3):611–619. doi: 10.1128/JVI.51.3.611-619.1984. PMID: 6088786.
16. Samulski RJ, Berns KI, Tan M, Muzyczka N. Cloning of adeno-associated virus into pBR322: rescue of intact virus from the recombinant plasmid in human cells. *Proc Natl Acad Sci USA.* 1982 Mar;79(6):2077–2081. doi: 10.1073/pnas.79.6.2077. PMID: 6281795.
17. Bulcha JT, Wang Y, Ma H, Tai PWL, Gao G. Viral vector platforms within the gene therapy landscape. *Signal Transduct Target Ther.* 2021 Feb 8;6(1):53. doi: 10.1038/s41392-021-00487-6. PMID: 33558455.
18. Ylä-Pelto J, Tripathi L, Susi P. Therapeutic use of native and recombinant enteroviruses. *Viruses.* 2016 Feb 23;8(3):57.
19. Rajawat YS, Humbert O, Kiem HP. In-vivo gene therapy with foamy virus vectors. *Viruses.* 2019 Nov 23;11(12):1091. doi: 10.3390/v11121091. PMID: 31771194.

# 14
# Early clinical gene therapy trials

By the early 1990s, not only were effective gene transfer vectors such as gammaretrovirus and adeno-associated virus (AAV) vectors suitable for human trials becoming available, but also the formal federal and local regulatory and review structures such as the National Institutes of Health (NIH) guidelines and *Points to Consider* and the RAC committee were in place to evaluate gene therapy proposals from the community. Furthermore, the gene therapy community was ready and anxious to move past the disastrous premature human clinical trials of beta-thalassemia gene therapy by Cline a decade earlier and begin to test a number of human disease models in clinical trials in real human patients. Steven Rosenberg and colleagues at the NIH were developing early approaches to immunotherapy of cancer and wished to understand the possible antitumor effects of apparently tumor-homing tumor-infiltrating lymphocytes (TIL) cells. They isolated TIL cells from a group of malignant melanoma patients, transduced them with a gammaretrovirus expressing a selectable neomycin-resistance gene marker and transfused the genetically modified cells back into the donor patients. The team found that the genetically modified cells survived in the patients' circulation and in patients' melanoma lesions for weeks to months, that the transduced cells demonstrated resistance to neomycin and that there was no detectable virus in the patients' circulation. There were no obvious adverse effects of the virus transfusions in the patients (1).

The study was more an early test of approaches to cancer immunotherapy than it was of gene therapy, but because it involved use of a virus vector to introduce a foreign gene into human beings, it was an important and successful test of the NIH and institutional gene therapy review mechanisms put into place after the Cline clinical trial and an important test of the recommendations of the 1982 President's commission and the NIH guidelines and *Points to Consider* for gene therapy studies. Even though it was not specifically a gene therapy study, it nevertheless demonstrated for the first time that a transgene could be introduced safely into human patients as a "marker" gene via transduced T-lymphocytes genetically modified with a gammaretrovirus vector.

Following closely on technical and administrative lessons learned from this first "marker" gene transfer study, William French Anderson and his NIH colleagues followed up on their preliminary research on a potential gene therapy for a form of severe combined immunodeficiency disease (SCID), a group of rare disorders characterized by defective development of a functional immune system with resulting susceptibility to life-threatening infections.*

Anderson and his group used a gammaretrovirus vector to transfer the wild-type human ADA cDNA (complementary DNA) into peripheral blood lymphocytes from two young patients with the adenosine deaminase (ADA) deficiency form of SCID (2). Until that time, the only treatments available for that lethal disease were multiple transfusions, enzyme-replacement therapy with polyethylene glycol–complexed ADA (PEG-ADA) and bone marrow transplantation, a treatment that is highly effective but that requires a well-matched bone marrow donor and carries significant morbidity and mortality. The NIH study was funded through a Cooperative Research and Development agreement (CRADA) that allows federal agencies like the NIH to establish joint programs with nonfederal institutions, in this case with the newly established biotech company Gene Therapy Inc. formed by Anderson specifically to produce their gene transfer vector for the gene therapy trial. As in many other areas of clinical research and even of early phase I clinical trials, evidence of positive clinical efficacy can often be implied in subtle ways even though phase I trials are designed to test safety and not clinical efficacy. In this early stage of gene therapy development, the interpretation of phase I gene therapy clinical trial goals and results were often described for the public and for the media as evidence of therapeutic breakthroughs. Such was the case with the early NIH ADA-SCID study.

In a follow-up evaluation of the two treated patients in 1995, the NIH group reported that both patients seemed to show clinical improvement with partly normalized cellular and humoral immune response and also that the integrated transduced ADA cDNA continued to be expressed. Apparently one patient was reported to show moderate restoration of ADA

---

* Kohn LA, Kohn DB. Gene therapies for primary immune deficiencies. *Frontiers in Immunology.* 2021;*12*:648951.

gene expression in 15% of her circulating lymphocytes, while the second patient demonstrated much lower ADA gene expression in a very low percent of circulating lymphocytes. Whether those levels of reconstituted ADA gene expression were sufficient to produce a long-term clinical improvement as claimed by the investigators is not fully clear, despite the frequent description of this clinical trial as the first successful human gene therapy study. Further complicating the interpretation of the trial is the fact that both patients had received treatments with a chemically stabilized formulation of the ADA enzyme known as PEG-ADA, a nongenetic treatment designed merely to add the missing ADA deaminase enzyme activity but not to correct the genetic defect.

Even in the absence of significant and rigorously convincing positive results, Anderson and his colleagues applied for patent protection for their procedures. Surprisingly and in a contentious decision, the U.S. Patent Office amazingly awarded the NIH a patent that applied to all ex vivo gene therapy studies in which genetic correction of cells is carried out in the laboratory followed by return of the genetically corrected cells to the patients to provide a new therapeutic source of the missing gene product. Fortunately, that patent decision has not impeded the use of the ex vivo model for gene therapy in the many subsequent studies over the following several decades to the present time. Interestingly, the investigators even applied for patent protection for in vivo gene therapy applications. That request was denied by the patent office.

Despite the fact that the study was frequently hyped in almost breathless terms as a therapeutic success, this trial gave evidence that the gene transfer tools and methods used were indeed safe and was therefore a successful phase I study. Even in the absence of convincing successful genetic correction, the study was also an important historical first test of the underlying concept of gene transfer technology and of the effectiveness of the NIH gene therapy oversight and review processes.

The enthusiasm for gene therapy grew following the reported success in the initial ADA study from the NIH group that generated misleadingly optimistic reports of impending gene therapy for other diseases, including cystic fibrosis, neurological diseases—even cancer (Figure 14.1). To some observers, these early attempts at human gene therapy were all being made to appear too easy through a combination of naiveté, well-intentioned wishful thinking, exaggerated published tentative results and possibly even a touch of hubris. There were even publications describing still early developing

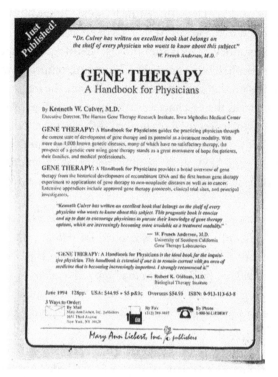

Figure 14.1. Marketing announcement for publication by Dr. Kenneth Culver in 1994 of a "physician's handbook" for gene therapy. This exemplifies the degree of exaggeration and hype surrounding the emerging field of gene therapy and contributed to the criticism of the field by the Orkin-Motulsky advisory committee to NIH Director Harold Varmus. Reproduced with permission from Mary Ann Liebert, Inc. Publishers.

complex technology as if it were ready for the practicing physician. It was not (See 1–4).

Subsequent ADA gene therapy studies were carried out with hematopoietic stem cells rather than peripheral blood lymphocytes. The use of those stem cells combined with preconditioning allowed more efficient and more stable correction of ADA expression in immune cell lineages. With those and subsequent additional modifications, gene therapy became established as the preferred therapeutic choice for this genetic disease.

As enthusiasm grew for extending gene therapy trials to additional disorders, some in the gene therapy community became uneasy about overblown interpretation and the hype of some early clinical results, such

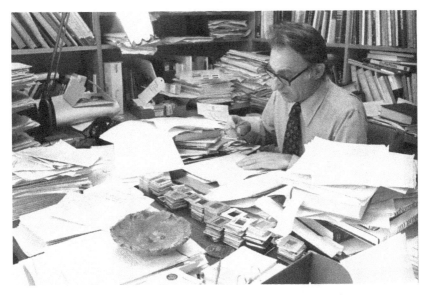

**Figure 14.2.** Arno Motulsky (1923–2018). German-American physician, human geneticist, molecular biology often described as a principal founder of human genetics and teacher to many in the field.

as those from the NIH SCID study, and about apparent absence of rigor in some of the preclinical studies (5). The concern grew so great that Harold Varmus, the director of the NIH, established an advisory committee chaired by a human clinical genetics founding father, Arno Motulsky (Figure 14.2) of the University of Washington, and Stuart Orkin (Figure 14.3) of Harvard University to examine the state of research and clinical activity in the field of gene therapy and to prepare a report that came to be entitled *Report and Recommendations of the Panel to Assess the NIH Investment in Research on Gene Therapy* (6).

Dr. Varmus had become alarmed that some of the research in the gene therapy field was shoddy and self-serving and suffered from "mistaken and widespread perception of success." The advisory committee recognized and supported the enormous potential benefits of gene therapy to medicine but concluded that the field of gene therapy had indeed gone astray and was badly in need of better preclinical and clinical research.

The Orkin-Motusky report concluded that, although the ultimate goals and aims of gene therapy were appropriate and worthy of support, the technology underlying gene therapy had been greatly hyped and oversold, that

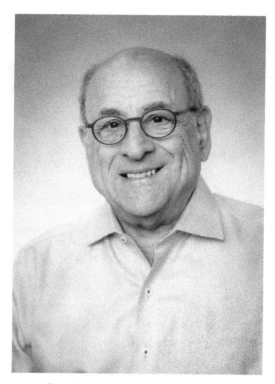

**Figure 14.3.** Stuart Orkin (b. 1946), physician and pediatric oncologist, molecular biologist at Harvard Medical School and Boston Children's Hospital. Courtesy of Stuart Orkin.

the NIH had been supporting too many clinical studies of little or no value and that the mechanisms of gene transfer needed to be better understood. The committee's findings were an unheard-of and serious public rebuke by national medical leadership of an important but errant developing area of biomedical research. The committee's message to the gene therapy community was unmistakable—get your house in order, improve the quality of your research and temper your rush to clinical trials. You are not yet ready for human clinical application.

### References

1. Rosenberg SA, Aebersold P, Cornetta K, Kasid A, Morgan RA, Moen R, Karson EM, Lotze MT, Yang JC, Topalian SL, et al. Gene transfer into humans—immunotherapy of patients with advanced melanoma, using tumor-infiltrating lymphocytes modified by retroviral gene transduction. *N Engl J Med*. 1990 Aug 30;323(9):570–578. doi: 10.1056/NEJM199008303230904.

2. Blaese RM, Culver KW, Chang L, Anderson WF, Mullen C, Nienhuis A, Carter C, Dunbar C, Leitman S, Berger M, et al. Treatment of severe combined immunodeficiency disease (SCID) due to adenosine deaminase deficiency with CD34+ selected autologous peripheral blood cells transduced with a human ADA gene. Amendment to clinical research project, Project 90-C-195, January 10, 1992. *Hum Gene Ther.* 1993 Aug;4(4):521–527. doi: 10.1089/hum.1993.4.4-521.
3. Flotte TR. Prospects for virus-based gene therapy for cystic fibrosis. *J Bioenerg Biomembr.* 1993 Feb;25(1):37–42. doi: 10.1007/BF00768066. PMID: 8382676 Review.
4. Hay JG, McElvaney NG, Herena J, Crystal RG. Modification of nasal epithelial potential differences of individuals with cystic fibrosis consequent to local administration of a normal CFTR cDNA adenovirus gene transfer vector. *Hum Gene Ther.* 1995 Nov;6(11):1487–1496. doi: 10.1089/hum.1995.6.11-1487. PMID: 8573621 Clinical Trial.
5. Friedmann T. Rigor in gene therapy studies. *Gene Ther.* 1995 Aug;2(6):355–356.
6. Orkin SH, Motulsky AG. Report and recommendations of the panel to assess the NIH investment in research on gene therapy, Report to the NIH Director. *Bull Med Ethics.* 1996 March;116:10–11.

# 15

# From academia to the bedside—the design of clinical trials

With the inexorable academic scientific progress in gene transfer technology, the field of gene therapy was faced with the problem of learning how best to deliver these complicated and astounding techniques efficiently and affordably to real patients with real disease. Gene therapy found itself confronted by all of the logistical and ethical dilemmas facing all forms of human clinical and experimental research.

The modern gold standard for human clinical studies has been established during the latter half of the 20th century by the concept of randomized clinical trials (RCT). Such an approach is not entirely new in medicine and certainly predates even the Hippocrates dictum, "do no harm." In fact, human clinical trials can trace their origin as far back as the 6th century BC during the reign of the Babylonian king Nebuchadnezzar (Figure 15.1) (1). At one time during his reign, the mad and grass-eating Babylonian king ordained that his subjects were required to eat only meat and drink only wine. However, some of his royal subjects objected and chose to continue their diet of legumes and water. The king relented and allowed them a short period of ten days to follow their preferred diet. At the end of the short "trial," the king concluded that his bean-eating subjects seemed to be in better health, and therefore the meat and wine mandate was rescinded.

A more recognizably modern and probably the first true clinical trial was described in 1753 in a paper entitled "*A Treatise on the Scurvy*" by the English naval physician James Lind. Lind had divided his ship's crew into 12 groups of two sailors each and treated them with a variety of substances including barley water, sea water, vinegar and, in one group, oranges and lemons. Only the two sailors who had been receiving oranges and lemons remained well, while the others developed scurvy. Thus came the end of the experiment and the origin of the English term "limey" for British sailor (2).

During the 19th and 20th centuries, concepts of the design of clinical trials in medicine became more established and codified. In 1966, Henry Beecher

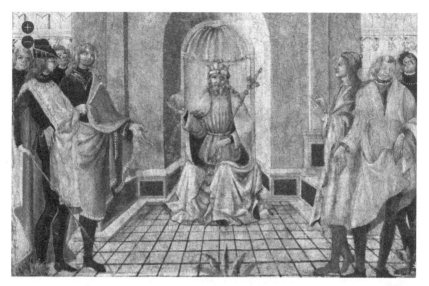

**Figure 15.1.** Nebuchadnezzar (630–561 BC), second king of the Neo-Babylonian empire. Courtesy of the Metropolitan Museum of Art.

of Harvard University cited multiple examples of unethical practices in clinical research and summarized the conditions under which clinical research could legitimately be done (3). His work was foundational in the history of all clinical research. He laid greater emphasis on professional "carelessness" and the need in human clinical studies for virtuous self-scrutiny rather than regulation.

Beecher's work came in the shadow of several technically and ethically disastrous human clinical studies/experiments that sadly did much to spur on the development of legitimate human clinical studies. Those scientific and ethical transgressions included the involuntary sterilization of "unfit" humans as endorsed by the U.S. Supreme Court in its infamous 1927 *Buck v. Bell* decision (4), the horrors of the Nazi medical experimentation programs during World War II (5), the misguided Tuskegee syphilis experiment by the U.S. Public Health Service in which black syphilis patients were denied curative penicillin treatment for the purpose of understanding the natural history of the disease (6), the American hepatitis experiment in which institutionalized retarded children at the Willowbrook State Institution in New Jersey were deliberately infected with hepatitis virus in order to allow the investigators to track the epidemiology of the disease (7).

How and why did those experimental "studies" fail many of the existing requirements for good science? The requirements for ethically acceptable application of emerging technologies to human subjects were defined and promulgated in a variety of international declarations, most notable among them being the Nuremberg Code in 1947, the Helsinki Declaration of 1964 (8), the Belmont report issued in 1976 by the U.S. National Commission for the Protection of Human Subjects of Biomedical and Behavioral Research (9). Interestingly, coincident with the Nuremberg trials, one of the very first blinded and randomized control clinical trials was carried out in 1947 by Geoffrey Marshall at the Medical Research Council in England to determine the efficacy of streptomycin on the treatment of tuberculosis.

The ethical principles essential for all human experimentation established and codified by those declarations included the requirement for informed consent and autonomy by research subjects and the requirements that a clinical study be designed in the best interest of subjects (beneficence), by the Hippocratic dictum of not doing harm (nonmaleficence) and the requirement for justice and fairness for research subjects. Without doubt, the legalized involuntary sterilization programs endorsed by the U.S. Supreme Court, the Cline gene therapy study, the Tuskegee syphilis study, the Willowbrook hepatitis study and others should all have failed to live up to those requirements. Although early gene therapy studies such as the initial NIH (National Institutes of Health) SCID (severe combined immunodeficiency disease) gene therapy experiment and several other exaggerated claims of imminent gene therapy treatments for diseases such as cystic fibrosis did comply with existing ethical constraints, they were marred by the tendency of investigators to raise false hopes, as noted by the advisory committee to the NIH director Harold Varmus in its unprecedented rebuke of the field of gene therapy in 1995.

As the concepts and tools of gene therapy matured with increasing speed and as more and more preclinical studies demonstrated proof of concept in the last decade of the 20th century and the beginning of the 21st century, the gene therapy community, especially in the United States and in Europe was spurred on by a palpable and almost urgent sense of optimism that the time was ripe for well-designed clinical trials. Most early studies were phase I studies designed ostensibly merely to test the safety of an agent, although there was often a sense of expectation of clinical efficacy. Increasingly, more mature studies were designed as phase II and even randomized clinical phase III trials (10) intended to evaluate efficacy in comparison to other existing therapies and eventually to lead to licensing and approval for public use by the regulatory agencies such as the Food and Drug Administration (FDA) and European Medicines Agency (EMA) for public use. The gene therapy community clearly understood the requirements of clinical trial design and had learned from the setbacks and errors in early-stage studies such as the Cline and early NIH SCID studies that true convincing clinical success would come only through rigorous science and with careful adherence to rigorous tenets of ethical design of clinical trials.

## References

1. Oberbaum M, Lysy J, Gropp C. From Nebuchadnezzar to the randomized controlled trial—milestones in the development of clinical research. *Harefuah.* 2011 Aug;150(8):668–671, 686.
2. Bhatt A. Evolution of clinical research: a history before and beyond James Lind. *Perspect Clin Res.* 2010 Jan;1(1):6–10.
3. Beecher HK. Ethics and clinical research. *N Engl J Med.* 1966 Jun 16;274(24):1354–1360. doi: 10.1056/NEJM196606162742405.
4. Silver MG. Eugenics and compulsory sterilization laws: providing redress for victims of a shameful era in United States history. *George Washington Law Rev.* 2004 Apr;72(4):862–892.
5. Thieren M, Mauron A. Nuremberg code turns 60. *Bull World Health Organ.* 2007 Aug;85(8):573. doi: 10.2471/blt.07.045443.
6. Rothman DJ, Were Tuskegee & Willowbrook 'studies in nature'? *Hastings Cent Rep.* 1982 Apr;12(2):5. PMID: 7096065.
7. Khuroo MS, Sofi AA. The discovery of hepatitis viruses: agents and disease. *J Clin Exp Hepatol.* 2020 Jul-Aug;10(4):391–401. doi: 10.1016/j.jceh.2020.04.006. Epub 2020 Apr 20. PMID: 32655240.
8. Shrestha BM. The Declaration of Helsinki in relation to medical research: historical and current perspectives. *J Nepal Health Res Counc.* 2012 Sep;10(22):254–257. PMID: 23281462 Review.
9. Adashi EY, Walters LB, Menikoff JA. The Belmont Report at 40: reckoning with time. *Am J Public Health.* 2018 Oct;108(10):1345–1348. doi: 10.2105/AJPH.2018.304580. Epub 2018 Aug 23. PMID: 30138058.
10. Kennedy HL. The importance of randomized clinical trials and evidence-based medicine: a clinician's perspective. *Clin Cardiol.* 1999 Jan;22(1):6–12. doi: 10.1002/clc.4960220106.

# 16

# The Human Genome Project—a complement, but not the origin, of gene therapy

In parallel with the advances during the 1980s and 1990s in virology, gene transferring methods, computing technology, knowledge of the genetic basis of human disease and awkward early gene therapy trials, it was inevitable that the DNA sequencing tools developed by Fred Sanger and Walter Gilbert would be applied to the most alluring target of all—the human genome. Despite the fact that by that time, the most important initial steps toward human gene therapy had already been taken—knowledge of disease models, development of gene transfer vectors, results of initial clinical trials—it was reasonable to think that elucidation of the entire human genome would add immense new power to gene therapy development, but even the most optimistic scientists realized that determining the sequence of the entire 3 billion bases of the human genome would require a brand new kind of "big science" effort. At that time, the most sophisticated tools had enabled determination of the nucleotide sequence of the genomes of only small mammalian and bacterial viruses—SV40, polyoma, PhiX174—consisting of no more that several thousand nucleotide base pairs of the genome.

That massive new technological and logistical effort came beginning in 1988 in the form of the Human Genome Project—an entirely new way to do big science. In 1985, Robert Sinsheimer convened a workshop at the University of California Santa Cruz to determine approaches to applying the newly established DNA sequencing technology to establish a complete human reference genome sequence. The idea of fully sequencing the human genome and giving it some potential financial credibility was endorsed by Charles DeLisi and David Smith of the U.S. Department of Energy (DOE),

## 132  ORIGIN AND DEVELOPMENT OF GENETIC THERAPIES

Renato Dulbecco of the Salk Institute and by James Watson at the Cold Spring Harbor in New York. In 1988, the National Institutes of Health (NIH) formally established its Human Genome Program under the directorship of James Watson of DNA double helix fame, and in 1990 the NIH, under its new director Francis Collins, and the DOE coordinated their plans to initiate the Human Genome Project with $3 billion funding. The Project established a broad international coalition of more than 2000 investigators in interactive centers in the United States, England, Germany, France and Japan toward the goal of defining the genetic, physical and complete nucleotide maps of the human genome and that committed participating centers to completely open and immediate access of all data. Such a massive, interactive and open research project defined a new approach to biological research and also committed 5% of its annual budget to the ethical, legal and social issues associated with the sometimes-contentious goals of completely determining the nucleotide sequence of the human genome.

In 1998, Craig Venter, CEO of the firm Celera Genomics, initiated a privately funded total human genome sequencing program that would proceed

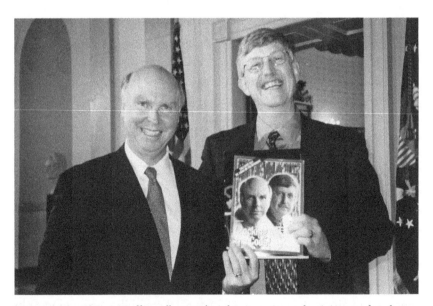

**Figure 16.1.** Francis Collins, (b. 1950) right. American physician, molecular biologist and director of the U.S. National Institutes of Health (2009–2021) and John Craig Venter (b. 1946) left, American molecular biologist and geneticist, celebrating the publication by the international consortium of the initial draft of the human genome DNA sequence in 2000.

in parallel with the NIH-DOE program with somewhat different patenting and data sharing policies and, with $300 million, a much lower cost than the publicly funded NIH-DOE program. Eventually, the two parallel programs simultaneously published preliminary >80% drafts of their sequence results, and by December 2022, the sequence of the human genome was nearly 100% completely determined.

While the Human Genome Project was an immense success at establishing a completely new approach to an international consortium for solving very big problems in biology, and while mapping techniques emerging from the project identified many new disease models potentially amenable to gene-based therapies, it added very little major new strength to the concepts and tools of human gene therapy. The Human Genome Project and advances in gene therapy therefore were independent, parallel and only partly complementary adventures in the remarkable modern era of biomedical science. More impressively, the completion of the Human Genome Project represented not merely the delivery of a scientific promise and the culmination of centuries of descriptive genetics but, more importantly, the first glimpse into a new era of redesigning human biology (Figure 16.1).

# 17
# A third serious setback

The gene therapy community took to heart the criticisms and recommendations of the Orkin-Motulsky NIH (National Institutes of Health) advisory committee and the negative press accounts of the breathless exaggeration that characterized some of the initial gene therapy studies. The period from 1995 until 1999 was characterized more by a heads-down determination to make the basic and preclinical progress that would be necessary for designing and implementing truly effective clinical trials. Gone, at least quiescent, was the overly enthusiastic and self-promoting hyperbole of the previous few years and basic and preclinical research proceeded. Yes—there certainly was enthusiasm but it took the form of more understated and quiet optimism, not exactly like the severe "hype" of the previous decade.

One of the most promising clinical gene therapy trials during that time involved an adenovirus-based trial of gene therapy for the X-linked liver-based urea cycle disorder ornithine transcarbamylase (OTC) deficiency characterized by life-threatening hyperammonemia and resulting in metabolic derangement, developmental delay, intellectual disabilities, and other multiple neurological symptoms such as ataxia, seizures and psychiatric symptoms. The genetic defect leads to defective protein metabolism and elevated levels of ammonia. The severity of symptoms varies with the age of onset, with the most severe symptoms in the neonatal and early childhood ages. Late onset both in males and females can be associated with less severe symptoms, but all patients, whether severe or mild, are susceptible to acute episodes of hyperammonemia.

Treatment for acute symptoms of OTC deficiency classically involves nitrogen scavenging with phenylbutyrate and L-citrulline, reversal of catabolism, dietary restriction of protein intake and supplementation with essential amino acids. In severe cases, as in neonatal patients, the most definitive treatment is liver transplantation.

Jesse Gelsinger was an 18-year-old, reasonably healthy OTC patient who was being fairly successfully managed and stabilized with standard dietary therapy despite having a history of hyperammonemic episodes (Figure 17.1).

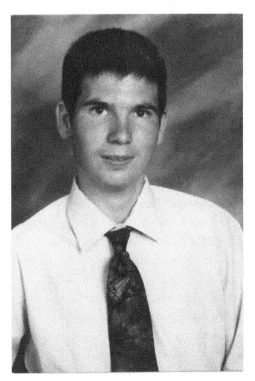

**Figure 17.1.** Jesse Gelsinger (1981–1999), at his high school graduation and later a patient in the University of Pennsylvania gene therapy clinical trial of ornitihine transcarbamylase deficiency. Courtesy of Dr. Paul Gelsinger.

He learned about a clinical gene therapy trial being conducted for OTC deficiency at the University of Pennsylvania by the eminent metabolic disease physician Mark Batshaw and the director of the gene therapy, James Wilson (Figure 17.2). There were few, if any, institutions where this kind of study might have succeeded. The university's gene therapy program was certainly one of the very best in the country, very well-funded with millions of dollars in research support, and directed by Dr. Wilson, considered by many, according to his NIH colleague French Anderson, to be first rate and, according to Anderson, "present company excluded, he's the best person in the field."

Up until that time, Jesse had been treated with dietary restriction therapy, but he had experienced a number of serious metabolic crises during his life. He, his family and his doctors all hoped for a more healthful life through gene therapy. The clinical trial involved direct injection into the portal vein

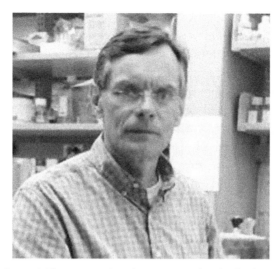

Figure 17.2. James Wilson, America physician, molecular biologist and director of the University of Pennsylvania Gene Therapy Center carrying out the clinical gene therapy trial of ornithine transcarbamylase in which Jesse Gelsinger was enrolled. Courtesy of Sabina Louise Pierce

that leads into the liver of an adenovirus vector expressing the normal OTC cDNA (complementary DNA). Preliminary studies by the Penn group had reported correction of the liver defect in OTC-deficient mice, and they had also carried out toxicity studies in monkeys. Based on their experience, the Penn group sought and received approval from their university's human subjects and biosafety committees for a human clinical trial in OTC patients. Their proposal was to conduct a phase I trial, meaning that it was intended to establish safety and not clinical efficacy. The study was an important component of the University of Pennsylvania's largely successful commitment to establish the world's most important premier gene therapy center. It reflected the laudable exuberance of the investigators and their university to be recognized as inventors of this new field of medicine. Governmental regulators encouraged the rapid transfer of biomedical advances to the public welfare, and the rapidly growing biotech industry was anxious to profit from the technology of gene-based therapy, and in the case of Wilson's own company Genovo, Inc., provided major funding for the trial of Batshaw and Wilson, positioning themselves to become leaders in driving this new field of medicine to the marketplace and potentially to reap large financial rewards.

Before his involvement with gene therapy, Jesse Gelsinger was in relatively stable metabolic health and was being controlled by his life-long medical support with many medications for amino acid and general metabolic stabilization and for normalized liver function. Despite this treatment he, like many other OTC patients, suffered episodes of dangerous and even life-threatening hyperammonemia. But he and his family wished for a more normalized teenage life, and as is true of most participants in human clinical studies, Jesse's motivation was based on a mixture of a hope for a better life for himself and also an altruistic wish for a normal life for other OTC patients.

Jesse was accepted into the Penn OTC clinical trial and was placed into a later cohort of patients who previously had apparently successfully gone through their treatment procedure. Very shortly after he received his injection of the adenovirus vector injection, Jesse suffered a severe immune response, a "cytokine storm" that caused widespread intravascular bleeding and generalized organ failure. Jesse died on the fourth day of his trial (1).

Jesse's death was a disaster and crushing loss of course to the Gelsinger family. It also dealt a very great blow to the Penn gene therapy team and to the field of gene therapy as a whole. Investigations of the cause of Jesse's death revealed multiple alarming technical and procedural deficits and errors by the investigators, including failure of the investigators to take adequate note of serious potentially harmful results and several deaths in their prior monkey studies, adverse reactions in preceding patients, pre-injection test results for Jesse that might have predicted serious harmful immune response or even excluded him from progressing to further stages of the study. To add to these problems, the study was found by NIH, FDA and University of Pennsylvania investigative committees to be flawed by a serious conflict of interest on Dr. Wilson's part stemming from his role as a decision-maker in the Philadelphia biotech firm Genovo Inc. that he founded and that was providing major funding for the Penn clinical trial and in which Wilson had a very large financial interest. The investigators also identified troubling ethical lapses and oversights in Jesse's consent forms and failure to notify Jesse and his family of serious adverse events in some of their animal studies using similar materials and methods.

As a result of the multiple investigations and the resulting legal suits, the NIH halted its grant support for the study, the university disbanded its gene therapy program, and Dr. Wilson was prohibited by the FDA from taking part in future clinical gene therapy trials. The overall experience underscored the danger of somewhat flawed preclinical studies in an experimental new field of medicine and the instances of inadequate attention paid to ethical and technical warning signals. While technical misjudgments and ethical lapses by Dr. Wilson and clinical associates were judged by all of the investigative committees to lie at the heart of the clinical disaster, the exuberant aura of optimism and expectation for a major scientific medical and commercial success that permeated the gene therapy institute at the University of Pennsylvania may have allowed a degree of institutional laxity in designing the academic and commercial collaboration supporting the clinical trial. But the central decision-making role that Wilson played in the disastrous clinical trial was underscored when, almost a decade later, Wilson published his personal partial accounting of the institutional and personal lapses contributing to the failure of the clinical trial (2).

The death of Jesse Gelsinger and the dismantling of what was considered by many at the time to be the country's, and even one of the world's premier gene therapy programs, was an enormous disaster to the field of gene therapy. Scientific criticism was harsh, and public and press commentary was unforgiving. There was a palpably deep sense of despair during that year's annual meeting of the American Society of Gene Therapy. A feeling of "were we on the wrong track" seemed to prevail just at a time when so much excellent and well-designed research was being presented at the meeting and when, looking more dispassionately into the future, success was inevitable. Many saw the OTC experience as the third in the series of severe gene therapy setbacks following the Martin Cline studies at UCLA in 1980, and the harsh rebuke of the quality of research in the field by the NIH director and his advisory committee in 1995. There was serious doubt if and how the concept and the field of gene therapy could recover from this most serious setback. Was the field of gene therapy nothing more than self-promoting hyperbole built on inadequate science? What the field of gene therapy desperately needed was credible clinical successes, and fortunately, the gene therapy community had, like Dr. Wilson, learned crucial lessons about the technical and ethical design of gene therapy clinical trials. Based on those lessons and rapid advancement in technology, successes were about to appear.

### References

1. Couzin J, Kaiser J. As Gelsinger case ends, gene therapy suffers another blow. *Science.* 2005;307(5712):1028. https://www.science.org/doi/10.1126/science.307.5712.1028b
2. Wilson JM. Lessons learned from the gene therapy trial for ornithine transcarbamylase deficiency. *Mol Genet Metab.* 2009 Apr;96(4):151–157. doi: 10.1016/j.ymgme.2008.12.016. Epub 2009 Feb 10. PMID: 19211285.

# 18
# Finally—breakthrough success?

Following the disastrous failure of the Penn OTC (ornithine transcarbamylase) gene therapy trial, the first decade of the 21st century was kinder to the field of gene therapy and provided much-needed good news. Important studies were illuminating the mechanisms underlying the earlier clinical failures for OTC deficiency and other preliminary clinical trials, but more importantly, they demonstrated credible clinical successes for several diverse human genetic diseases. What led to the clinical gene therapy advances and even clinical successes was a combination of better science, better design of clinical trials and the maturation of the powerful pharma and biotech activities that contributed to the technological maturation of the field but also came to be the major catalyst for driving the clinical phases of gene therapy. Academia excels in innovation and research, but it is usually inadequately prepared to implement novelties and to deliver them to broad public use. That is the area of expertise and experience of the pharmaceutical industry and, especially in the case of gene therapy, the emerging role of new, often start-up biotechnology firms that have led the way to clinical application but also to research advances. Increasingly, standard academia has come to take a back seat in the field.

These early clinical studies and clinical trials were largely based on the conceptually straightforward approach of adding new therapeutic genetic information to take the place of a genetic defect—an approach to therapy inherent in Archibald Garrod's concept of inborn errors of metabolism. The most straightforward concept flowing from Garrod's work is that treatment of a genetic disease, at least an inborn error of metabolism, could be achieved by augmenting a disease-related genome with a normal copy of the aberrant gene responsible for disease, rather than correcting the underlying disease gene. Of course, it was not possible in those early days of gene therapy to foresee ways in which disease-causing genes could be replaced or even have their genetic mutations corrected; i.e., by methods of genome "editing" that were to become feasible several decades later. That kind of change of the spelling of the human genome and of disease-causing genes has long been dreamt about but was considered out of reach. Many had imagined the eventual development of such methods in the far distant future, but very few scientists were prepared for the speed with which that genetic manipulative technology came upon human genetics at the beginning of the 21st century.

In China, a large clinical trial was conducted by the gene therapy biotechnology firm Shenzhen SiBiono GeneTech Co. Ltd., with an adenovirus vector product called *Gendicine* expressing a wild-type complementary DNA (cDNA) for the well-recognized prototypical cancer surveillance tumor suppressor gene p53. The p53 gene is known to be mutated in a high percentage of human cancers and is recognized as the immediate cause of the human cancer disease Li-Fraumeni Syndrome characterized by multiple tumors. Its importance as a tumor suppressor gene has supported the concept that restoration of wild-type p53 function in cancer cells by a virus vector–transduced p53 transgene might reverse aspects of the tumor phenotype. As a result of very large preliminary human clinical trials reporting clinical efficacy in a variety of cancers, especially head and neck cancers, an adenovirus expressing wild-type p53 received approval in 2003 for commercialization from the Chinese State Food and Drug Administration (CSFDA), thereby becoming the world's first formally licensed gene therapy product. It was reported to lead to many successful instances of progression-free clinical responses, justifying its approved in 2003 by the China Food and Drug Administration (CFDA) for treatment of head and neck cancer. In 2004, Gendicine thereby became the first in-class gene therapy product to enter the commercial market, almost entirely in China.

In fact, the concept and the design of the *Gendicine* study was similar to an adenovirus-vector cancer therapy platform being developed in the United States, but progress in those latter studies was slow and insufficiently convincing to receive FDA approval. One such adenovirus-based agent, *Advexin,* was developed by the American biotech company Introgen, but it was rejected for clinical approval by the American Food and Drug Administration (FDA) in 2008 and was also withdrawn for consideration by the European Medicines Administration (EMA). While these adenovirus-based cancer gene therapy agents may have held, and may still hold, some clinical promise, they did not provide the rescue that the field of gene therapy was looking for.

Several additional positive results were reported in gene therapy studies and approved in China, Russia and the Philippines. A follow-up adenovirus-based gene therapy aimed at head and neck cancer was approved in China in 2005. A gammaretrovirus Rexin-G was approved in 2007 in the Philippines for cancer gene therapy, and a plasmid-based vector approach was developed by the Human Stem Cells Institute in Russia to introduce the vascular endothelial growth factor (VEGF) into arteries of patients with peripheral artery disease.

Unlike the disastrous results with the adenovirus vectors in OTC deficiency and the unconfirmed results with the adenovirus vector *Gendicine* in the Chinese gene therapy studies for cancer, more promising results were emerging in several independent gene therapy trials for two different forms of primary severe combined immunodeficiency disease (SCID)—the same set of diseases proposed for gene therapy by French Anderson and his NIH (National Institutes of Health) colleagues a decade earlier. Most impressively and at the same time, very promising results were emerging from a gene therapy trial conducted by a Paris-London-based gene therapy group headed by the immunologist-physician Alain Fischer in an experimental treatment for the X-linked form of SCID. Clinically, X-linked SCID is similar to the ADA-deficiency immune disease studied by Anderson and his NIH colleagues in the early 1990s. The only known truly effective treatment for this disorder was bone marrow transplantation with marrow from a donor sibling or even from an unrelated donor. As an attractive model system for gene therapy, SCID had become a rather famous disease because of the saga of David Vetter, a boy born at Texas Children's Hospital in 1971 in Houston who had been identified by prenatal diagnosis to have X-linked SCID (see Figure 18.1). Mere seconds after his birth he was taken to a sealed tent designed by NASA aeronautical engineers where he lived for most of his short life. In 1983 his doctors attempted to treat him by bone marrow transplantation, but the procedure failed, and several months after the transplant, David died of a lymphoma, possibly the consequence of the marrow transplantation procedure. David Vetter became known world-wide as the "Texas bubble boy."

As early as 1999, Alain Fischer at the Necker Hospital in Paris (Figure 18.2) and colleagues at the Great Ormond Hospital for Children in London had been independently developing a clinical trial involving a murine leukemia virus (MLV)-based gammaretrovirus expressing the wild-type cDNA

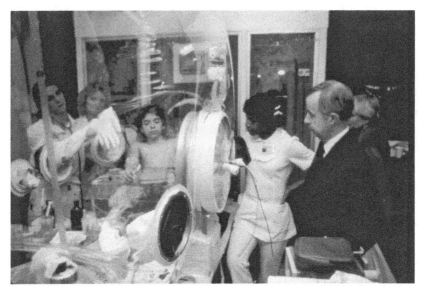

**Figure 18.1.** David Vetter (1971–1984), the "Texas bubble-boy" diagnosed at birth to be afflicted with severe combined immunodeficiency disease (SCID). Courtesy of the Baylor College of Medicine Archives.

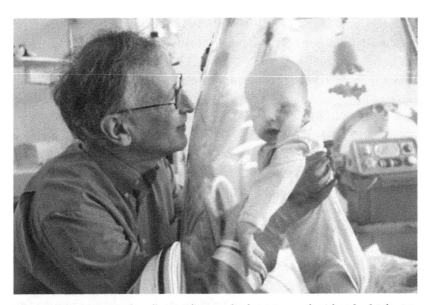

**Figure 18.2.** Alain Fischer (b. 1949), French physician and molecular biologist shown in 2002 treating a patient in his SCID gene therapy trial. Reproduced with kind permission from Alain Fischer.

for the gene responsible for the disease—the gene that encodes the cytokine receptor subunit common to interleukins IL-2, IL-4, IL-7, IL-9, IL-15 and IL-21. The developmental defect of those vital cytokines leads to complete failure of both T and NK lymphocyte immune cell lineages and resulting immunodeficiency. By 2002, Fischer, Marina Cavazzano and their combined Paris–London team had treated a total of 20 children (1), all of whom lacked an HLA-(human leukocyte antigens)-identical sibling or other potentially suitable donors to allow attempts at bone marrow transplantation therapy. Of those 20 patients, 17 showed an extraordinary, stable and very broad correction of their immune deficits for up to 13 years, and most of the children seemed to be on their way to a normal childhood life (2). Several of the children showed less robust and only partial immune reconstitution. Nevertheless, this remarkable result seemed to be the first demonstration of a significant clinical success in a gene therapy trial. SCID was emerging as a superb model system for establishing methods for human gene therapy. Finally, the field of gene therapy seemed to have received some good news.

Sadly, that initial optimism was dealt a serious blow when, in 2003, the Paris group announced that at first one, and then eventually a total of five treated children who had shown early therapeutic early immune reconstitution subsequently developed very similar cases of T-cell acute lymphoblastic leukemia between 2 and 5 years after the gene therapy procedure. One child died of that disease, and the other four responded to leukemia treatment and survived. There was obviously a fatal flaw in the design of the therapeutic protocol. The French and English officials as well as the NIH immediately put SCID clinical gene therapy trials on hold until the cause of the leukemias could be established. Very quickly, an international group of gene therapy investigators confirmed that the leukemias were a direct result of the gene transfer technology. It was shown that the transducing MLV-based vector had integrated near the quiescent protooncogene LMO2, but the integration event activated LMO2 expression and, together with induced mutations in several other genes including *NOTCH1*, deletion of the tumor suppressor gene cyclin-dependent kinase 2A (*CDKN2A*), and translocation of the TCR-β region to the *STIL-TAL1* locus, the combination of those multiple disruptive events had activated neoplastic mechanisms in the cells. The long-suspected potential problem of insertional mutagenesis genotoxicity by retrovirus vectors in human gene therapy had tragically come to pass in this gene therapy study.

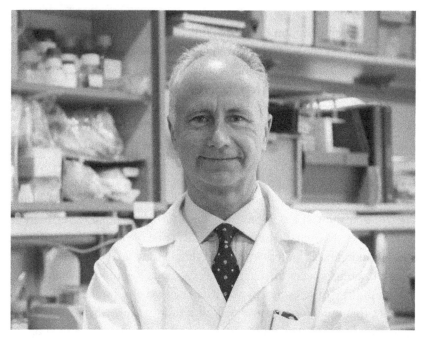

**Figure 18.3.** Allessandro Aiuti (b. 1966), Italian physician, molecular biologist and gene therapy investigator and major contributor to genetic therapy of SCID and other primary immunodeficiencies. Reproduced with kind permission from Alessandro Aiuti.

Just as these problems of harmful effects of genetic modification of the genome ("genotoxicity") were becoming recognized for the use of a gammaretrovirus in X-SCID, several groups, particularly the groups of Allesandro Aiuti (Figure 18.3), Luigi Naldini and Claudio Bordignon at the San Raffaele Hospital in Milan were finding far fewer problems with their use of a conceptually similar but technically improved approach to gene therapy for the exact disease model that had previously been studied by Anderson and Blaese and the NIH group in 1992; i.e., the immunodeficiency disease caused by mutations of the gene encoding adenosine deaminase. In contrast to the use in the NIH trial of peripheral lymphocytes as targets for genetic correction, the Milan groups led by Aiuti chose to use the gammaretrovirus vector to target bone marrow CD34+ hematopoietic stem cells instead of peripheral blood lymphocytes and to include low-dose myeloablation preparation of patients to make their bone marrow spaces receptive to the genetically corrected CD34+ cells (2). Those changes to the earlier Anderson approach in the NIH study made all the difference in the world.

After treatment, the majority of their ADA-SCID patients showed high levels of engraftment of the genetically corrected cells, normalized ADA gene expression, immune reconstitution, and normalized T-cell numbers and T-cell function. Furthermore, their patients no longer required enzyme-replacement therapy and were able to resume a largely normalized childhood lifestyle free of adventitious infections. These and similar results from additional gene therapy groups have established gene therapy as a safe and effective treatment for ADA-SCID, even establishing what might become a new standard of care for that disease (3). The methodology used for this study was the basis for a commercially available product called *Strimvelis* developed by the Milan-based biotech firm MolMed in collaboration with the pharmaceutical company GlaxoSmithKline (GSK). Despite its obvious effectiveness and its advantages over enzyme replacement and over the previous gene therapy approach proposed in 1992 by French Anderson and his NIH team, *Strimvelis* had become a commercial problem because of its very high price (approximately $1 million) in the face of dearth of suitable numbers of patients and because of the development of leukemia in one patient, reminiscent of the serious adverse events encountered in the X-SCID studies of Fischer and his colleagues in 2002. As a result, *Strimvelis* was removed from the market.

Similar approaches have subsequently been extended to develop gene-based therapies for other primary immunodeficiencies such as Wiskott-Aldrich Syndrome and chronic granulomatous disease (CGD) (4).

During the same period, equally remarkable successes were emerging from preclinical and clinical studies of still another inborn error of metabolism—the retinal degenerative disease Leber's congenital amaurosis (LCA), a group of autosomal recessive genetic disorders that are the most common cause of progressive blindness in infants and children. A group of geneticists and ophthalmologists including Gregory Acland at Cornell University, Jean Bennett at the University of Pennsylvania (Figure 18.4a) and William Hauswirth at the University of Florida and their colleagues were studying the Briard strain of dogs that suffers from a form of congenital blindness very similar to LCA. As in the human disease, the disease is caused by mutations of the RPE65 gene in the retinal pigmented epithelial cells of the retina that support the retinal photoreceptors. As early as 2001, they reported that they

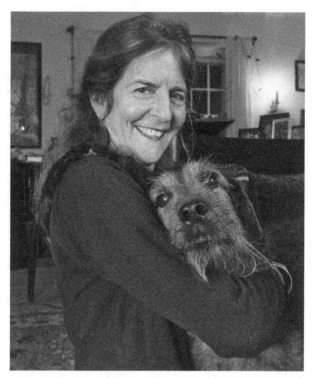

**Figure 18.4a.** Jean Bennett (b. 1954), American gene therapy investigator who pioneered AAV-mediated gene therapy for eye diseases such as Leber's Congenital Amaurosis.

successfully corrected the dog blindness disease and restored vision in the dogs with subretinal injections of a recombinant adeno-associated virus (AAV) vector expressing the wild-type RPE65 cDNA (5).

In 2008, the stunning success in dogs was then followed by the even more remarkable success with children with RPE65 LCA, one form of the 63 genetically distinct retinal disorders that cause blindness. Some, but not all, children who received subretinal injections of an AAV vector encoding the wild-type RPE65 cDNA demonstrated restoration of clinically useful vision (6), while adult patients showed smaller degrees and reduced durability of visual acuity and useful functional vision restoration (Figure 18.4b). This approach to the treatment of the LCA form of congenital blindness is obviously highly promising and is still undergoing extensive study to evaluate its durability and stability.

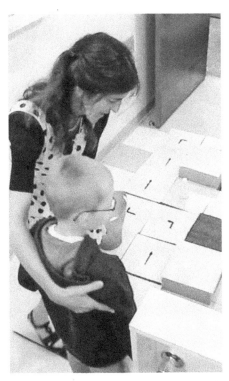

**Figure 18.4b.** Jean Bennett testing a treated patient with Leber's Congenital Amaurosis.

Additional impressive and startling successes for traditional, virus vector–mediated gene therapy came in 2019 with the development by Jerry Mendell (Figure 18.5) from the Ohio State University of an AAV-based therapy (Zolgesma) for the lethal neurodegenerative disease spinomuscular atrophy (SMA) caused by deficiency of the survival motor neuron (SMN1) gene (7). The disease causes progressive loss of muscle function and death. A major improvement in SMA treatment had earlier become available in 2016 with the development and FDA and EMA approval of the antisense oligonucleotide nusinersen that produced remarkable clinical improvement and prevented major disease progression. But its use was severely compromised by the need for frequent intrathecal injections. Zolgesma, approved by the FDA in 2019, offered major benefits over Spinraza, since it produced life-preserving neurological improvements but involved only a one-time intravenous injection of the AAV vector. The vector makes its way without specific targeting to the

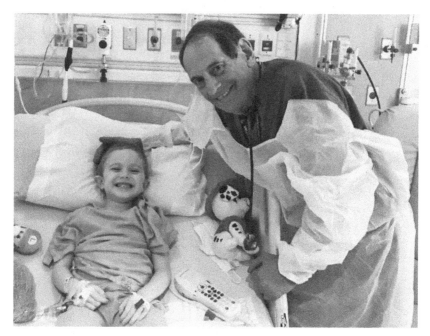

**Figure 18.5.** Jerry Mendell (b. 1942), American physician and gene therapy investigator, with interest in neurodegenerative diseases such as spinomuscular atrophy (SMA) and shown here examining a patient in a trial for gene therapy of Duchenne muscular atrophy. Courtesy of T. Friedmann.

liver where it integrates and produces therapeutic levels of SMN1 protein. This approach comes very close to being considered a "standard of care."

*Immunotherapy as gene therapy—CAR-T cells.* In addition to these impressive gene therapy results with monogenic inborn errors of metabolism, equally impressive therapeutic results have started to come in the case of more complex, probably multigenic disorders by manipulating the natural human host system that is designed to protect itself from onset of disease but that often fails to guard against the onset of malignant disease. We have come to learn that disease often results from the inability of the human immune system to prevent the onset of pathogenic events or to respond effectively to emerging disease. The advent of the concepts and techniques of gene therapy has suggested an entirely new approach to therapy of some very serious and often intractable forms of the blood cancers leukemia and lymphomas; i.e., to genetically redesign cells of the immune system to make them more responsive to pathogens or to pathogenic changes in cells and thereby create a new form of combined genetic- and immunotherapy.

Cancer in one form or other represents one of the most important target diseases for this kind of immunotherapy. It has long been known that a normal functional immune system is necessary for the prevention of cancer in humans and other mammals and that the surveillance function for detecting and suppressing emerging neoplastic cells is heavily mediated by T lymphocytes. The fact that the cancer surveillance system can and often does fail is documented by the fact that cancer does occur, alarmingly often. For reasons largely unknown, T cells lose their ability to recognize and home in on cancer cells and destroy them. Why and how does the T-cell surveillance mechanism fail, and could there be a genetic approach to restoring their function of targeting and killing cancer cells?

During the recent several decades a powerful correction for an ineffective immune system has been developed by genetic modification of T cells to express completely new synthetic chimeric receptors for tumor cell antigens (CAR) and thereby to allow the genetically modified T cells to recognize the surface molecules on cancer cells and restore the cancer cell–killing function to the cancer cells that had become invisible to immune surveillance. By this approach, genetic modification of a cancer-patient's autologous T cells and introduction of a gene encoding the synthetic CAR tumor cell receptor is performed by established viral or nonviral gene transfer methods as established for "traditional" gene therapy applications.

In 1987, Yoshikazu Kurosawa and his team in Japan reported that expression of an anti-phosphorylcholine chimeric receptor activated calcium influx in murine T-cell lymphoma EL4 cells when challenged with phosphorylcholine-positive bacteria, proving that a chimeric receptor could activate T cells in response to antigens (8).

In 1989 and 2001, Zelig Eshhar and his colleagues at the Weizmann Institute of Science in Israel (Figure 18.6) developed retrovirus-mediated gene transfer tools to express chimeric T-cell receptors, enabling the engineered T cells to seek out and destroy cancer cells that express the surface ligand molecules for the receptor (9).

This combined immunologic-genetic approach involving synthetic chimeric T-cell receptors has produced a revolutionary breakthrough for treatment of some forms of cancer, especially hematologic B-cell leukemias and lymphomas (10, 11). The clinical application of these concepts has been pursued by a number of laboratories, most notably that of Carl June at the

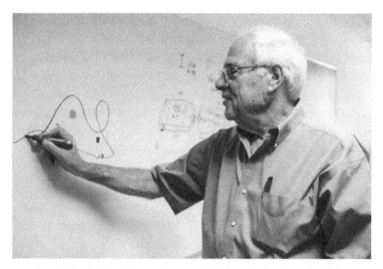

**Figure 18.6.** Zelig Eshhar (b. 1941), Israeli molecular biologist and cancer immunologist and pioneering investigator in CAR-T technology. Courtesy of Z Eshhar.

University of Pennsylvania (Figure 18.7). Eshhar and June shared the prestigious 2021 Dan David Prize.

Until the present time, the CAR-T approach to the treatment of cancer has been more effective for hematological malignancies, but many efforts are underway to extend the effectiveness of CAR-T immunotherapy to other cancers, including solid tumors that are refractory to effective therapy by current methods (11). To date, the extension of CAR-T immunotherapy to solid tumors has proven more difficult than for hematological malignancies, and success has been elusive. While this and other forms of immunotherapy are extremely promising and, when successful, lead to remarkable clinical responses, they suffer from a number of difficulties including severe toxicity, ineffective proliferation and shortened survival of the infused genetically modified CAR-T cells in patients, off-target trafficking and ineffective tumor cell infiltration, eventual loss of target antigen expression ("antigen escape") in tumor cells resulting in tumor relapse and, in common with other forms of gene-based therapies, their extremely high cost. Nevertheless, it is obvious that these problems are soluble and that immunotherapies are rapidly becoming major additions to chemotherapy and radiation therapy and other forms of cancer therapy.

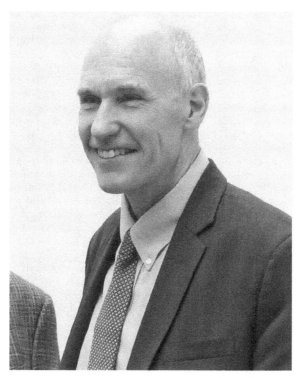

**Figure 18.7.** Carl June (b. 1953), American physician at the University of Pennsylvania and pioneering developer of CAR-T immunotherapy for cancer. Reproduced under Creative Commons Attribution-Share Alike 4.0 International license.

### References

1. Hacein-Bey-Abina S, Le Deist F, Carlier F, Bouneaud C, Hue C, De Villartay JP, Thrasher AJ, Wulffraat N, Sorensen R, Dupuis-Girod S, Fischer A, Davies EG, Kuis W, Leiva L, Cavazzana-Calvo M. Sustained correction of X-linked severe combined immunodeficiency by ex vivo gene therapy. *Engl J Med*. 2002 Apr 18;346(16):1185–1193. doi: 10.1056/NEJMoa012616.
2. Aiuti A, Cattaneo F, Galimberti S, Benninghoff U, Cassani B, Callegaro L, Scaramuzza S, Andolfi G, Mirolo M, Brigida I, Tabucchi A, Carlucci F, Eibl M, Aker M, Slavin S, Al-Mousa H, Al Ghonaium A, Ferster A, Duppenthaler A, Notarangelo L, Wintergerst U, Buckley RH, Bregni M, Marktel S, Valsecchi MG, Rossi P, Ciceri F, Miniero R, Bordignon C, Roncarolo MG. Gene therapy for immunodeficiency due to adenosine deaminase deficiency. *N Engl J Med*. 2009 Jan 29;360(5):447–458. doi: 10.1056/NEJMoa0805817.
3. Aiuti A, Roncarolo MG. Ten years of gene therapy for primary immune deficiencies. *Hematology Am Soc Hematol Educ Program*. 2009:682–689. doi: 10.1182/asheducation-2009.1.682. PMID: 20008254 Review.
4. Kohn LA, Kohn DB. Gene therapies for primary immune deficiencies. *Front Immunol*. 2021 Feb 25;12:648951. doi: 10.3389/fimmu.2021.648951. eCollection 2021. PMID: 33717203 Free PMC article.

5. Acland GM, Aguirre GD, Ray J, Zhang Q, Aleman TS, Cideciyan AV, Pearce-Kelling SE, Anand V, Zeng Y, Maguire AM, Jacobson SG, Hauswirth WW, Bennett J. Gene therapy restores vision in a canine model of childhood blindness. *Nat Genet.* 2001 May;28(1):92–95. doi: 10.1038/ng0501-92.
6. Maguire AM, Simonelli F, Pierce EA, Pugh EN Jr, Mingozzi F, Bennicelli J, Banfi S, Marshall KA, Testa F, Surace EM, Rossi S, Lyubarsky A, Arruda VR, Konkle B, Stone E, Sun J, Jacobs J, Dell'Osso L, Hertle R, Ma JX, Redmond TM, Zhu X, Hauck B, Zelenaia O, Shindler KS, Maguire MG, Wright JF, Volpe NJ, McDonnell JW, Auricchio A, High KA, Bennett J. Safety and efficacy of gene transfer for Leber's congenital amaurosis. *N Engl J Med.* 2008 May 22;358(21):2240–2248. doi: 10.1056/NEJMoa0802315. Epub 2008 Apr 27. PMID: 18441370.
7. Mendell JR, Al-Zaidy SA, Rodino-Klapac LR, Goodspeed K, Gray SJ, Kay CN, Boye SL, Boye SE, George LA, Salabarria S, Corti M, Byrne BJ, Tremblay JP. Current clinical applications of in vivo gene therapy with AAVs. *Mol Ther.* 2021 Feb 3;29(2):464–488. doi: 10.1016/j.ymthe.2020.12.007. Epub 2020 Dec 10. PMID: 33309881.
8. Kuwana Y, Asakura Y, Utsunomiya N, Nakanishi M, Arata Y, Itoh S, Nagase F, Kurosawa Y. Expression of chimeric receptor composed of immunoglobulin-derived V regions and T-cell receptor-derived C regions. *Biochem Biophys Res Commun.* 1987 Dec 31;149(3):960–968. doi: 10.1016/0006-291x(87)90502-x. PMID: 3122749.
9. Eshhar Z, Waks T, Bendavid A, Schindler DG. Functional expression of chimeric receptor genes in human T cells. *J Immunol Methods.* 2001 Feb 1;248(1–2):67–76. doi: 10.1016/s0022-1759(00)00343-4. PMID: 11223069.
10. June CH, O'Connor RS, Kawalekar OU, Ghassemi S, Milone MC. CAR T cell immunotherapy for human cancer. *Science.* 2018;359:1361–1365.
11. Sadelain M. $CD_{19}$ CAR T cells. *Cell.* 2017;171:1471.

# 19

# Gene editing—a foundational new era for genetic therapies

A new era of genetics has opened—one whose impact is comparable to the most epochal events in the history of science. It provides vivid proof for the observation of Sydney Brenner on how scientific progress is born; i.e., "Progress in science depends on new techniques, new discoveries and new ideas, probably in that order." In other words, technology is the major driving force for generating and enabling scientific progress—without new tools, advances in knowledge cannot move beyond dreams. This order of events has been the principle underlying the birth of a new kind of genetics that has already and will continue to completely reshape not only human gene therapy but every aspect of biology. It is called "gene editing."

Genetics is no longer a purely descriptive science, but rather has become a manipulative science. Not only are the mechanisms underlying the genetic basis of biological functions increasingly understood at a completely descriptive level, but the remarkable advances in biological science during the past century have demonstrated that genetic mechanisms can be manipulated to modify all aspects of the biological world and even to prevent and treat disease. Because the molecules and mechanisms of life are mostly, after all, chemicals of known structure, they are therefore amenable to chemical changes of forces that direct evolutionary change, driven not only by natural forces as discovered by Darwin, but also now by willful human intervention through designed modifications of the genomic targets of evolutionary change. Genetics has put power into human hands to alter and possibly even to define new directions of human biology and evolution.

During the first two decades of the 21st century, the direction to human gene therapy seems to have been irrevocably rerouted from an early phase of merely augmenting the genome with a therapeutic gene to the surprising new phase of rewriting the genome to edit the genetic spelling of disease-related functions. Genetics has arrived at an entirely revolutionary stage, previously only dreamt of. In contrast to the now "traditional" approaches to gene therapy—restoring genetic functions by augmenting the genome with "normal" forms of disease-related genetic functions, the continuing explosion of genetic technology has opened a conceptually new and astounding power for humanity to prevent and cure disease and even to shape its genetic future, with all of the promise and danger that such a power entails—for good and for ill.

Notwithstanding the explosive progress in manipulative genetics, the growing positive experience with vector-mediated transfer of therapeutic genes for gene therapy suggests that the "traditional" approach of virus-mediated gene transfer for gene therapy will for some time remain more amenable to gene-based therapies even in the face of the extremely exciting new era of more definitive gene and RNA editing, as described later in this chapter. The continued use of vector-mediated gene transfer approaches to therapy is underscored by the number and scope of European Medicines Agency (EMA)- and Food and Drug Administration (FDA)-approved clinical trials of gene transfer for treating both rare and common diseases including some forms of cancer, metabolic diseases, degenerative diseases such as osteoarthritis, and neurological disease. For instance, *bluebird bio* has recently received FDA and EMA approval for a lentivirus-mediated gene transfer product, Skysona (elivaldogene autotemcel), expressing the ABCD1 gene as an approach for gene therapy of the otherwise untreatable and fatal cerebral leukodystrophy. The Dutch biotech firm UniQure has reported development of a gene therapy approach for gene therapy of factor IX-deficiency hemophilia using a liver-targeted adeno-associated virus (AAV) vector called Hemgenix. These "classical" gene transfer methods for therapy are largely now with us, while clinical applications of genetic editing are in their earliest stages of infancy. But the startling and blindingly fast pace of progress in the new area of gene editing makes it evident that this approach will become the predominant gene therapy technology in the near future. The new era of genome editing will increasingly replace the current augmentation approaches to gene therapy with the concept of definitive editing-based correction of underlying causes of disease.

***Genome editing.*** Fortuitous advances in the unlikely field of microbial genetics are at the heart of this revolution and have led very rapidly to new and previously undreamed of applications in virtually every field of biological science. The traditional "classical" approach to human gene therapy, at least as it has evolved by the early 21st century, has generally been to augment the genome with elements to bypass pathogenic processes and thereby to restore normal genetic and physiological functions while accepting the continued presence in the corrected genome of the genetic aberrations responsible for disease. However, under the surface of that approach has been the hidden scientific wish not only to circumvent the mechanisms of pathogenesis but actually to edit and rewrite the genetic spelling of the sequences responsible for pathogenic mechanisms themselves. Until the latter part of the 20th century and the beginning of the 21st century, that goal has always seemed far beyond human grasp. It is no longer out of reach.

The most remarkable and least expected genetic breakthrough in the last several decades and the one with the greatest impact on gene therapy has been the development of methods to introduce targeted sequence changes into the genome and thereby to rewrite selected parts of the human genome. First tentative approaches toward that goal came in the mid-1980s when the laboratories of Oliver Smithies at the University of Wisconsin and the University of North Carolina and Mario Capecchi at the University of Utah developed recombinational methods to insert foreign sequences to specific sites and to target mutations in the human and murine genomes (1–3). For this work, Smithies and Capecchi shared the 2007 Nobel Prize in Physiology or Medicine. As exciting as those advances were at the time, the methods required powerful methods to select those rare cells carrying the altered genomes.

The prospect for more facile and even potentially therapeutic genome editing by rewriting the spelling of targeted pathogenic sequences exploded dramatically with the discovery of several endonucleases that in essence are restriction enzymes able to create double-strand breaks at any specified site in a target genome, breaks that then can be repaired by normal cellular mechanisms of non-homologous end joining (NHEJ) to create small mutations at a specific site—insertions or deletions (indels)—that serve to "knock out" or possibly to correct a resident sequence or, in the presence of an added template DNA, to insert or "knock-in" a novel sequence or transgene into the chromosome by homologous recombination (HR). These approaches to genome editing by targeted endonucleases have opened an astounding and conceptually new era of genetic science for research and therapeutic purposes. The most widely used of these endonucleases have been zinc finger nucleases, transcription activator-like (TAL) nucleases and clustered regularly interspaced short palindromic repeats (CRISPR) RNA-guided nucleases.

*Zinc finger endonucleases.* Zinc finger proteins are a large class of zinc-binding transcription factors discovered in 1985 by Aaron Klug at the MRC Laboratory of Molecular Biology (4). Rebar and Pabo (5) recognized in 1994 that the phage display system that they used to characterize zinc fingers provided a tool for studying protein–DNA interactions and "may offer a general method for selecting zinc finger proteins that recognize desired target sites on double-stranded DNA" and could direct DNA–protein interactions. That promise was fulfilled in 2007 by Srinivasan Chandrasegaran and his colleagues at Johns Hopkins University, who fused the nonspecific DNA cleavage domain of Fok I restriction endonuclease with a zinc finger to create the first truly targeted nuclease for producing site-specific double-strand breaks (DSB) to the genome (6). The broad application of Zn-finger genome editing was further documented in 2010 in a variety of eukaryotic target cells by F. Urnov and colleagues at Sangamo Therapeutics in San Francisco (7). The full potential power of Zn-finger editing was dramatically proven in 2014 by the use of Zn-finger nucleases to knock out the HIV receptors CCR5 and CXCR4 in human CD+ T cells, thereby making them resistant to infection with the HIV virus (8, 9), suggesting an approach to therapy and disease prevention.

The Zn-finger genome editing technology is currently being tested in multiple current human gene therapy clinical trials for several genetic diseases. One common clinical trial approach has been an in vivo process involving delivery of Zn-finger constructs into the human liver via the portal vein with the goal of inserting into the albumin locus of hepatocytes the wild-type genes of the factor IX gene for hemophilia B, the α-L-iduronidase (IDUA) gene for mucopolysaccharidosis type I, and iduronate 2-sulfatase (IDS) gene for mucopolysaccharidosis type II. In the case of the beta-thalassemia clinical trial, the ex vivo approach involved transducing CD34+ hematopoietic cells from patients with a Zn-finger construct that disrupts the BCL11A gene whose normal function is to suppress the expression of fetal hemoglobin (HbF) in erythrocytes. Restored elevated expression of HbF is known to substitute functionally for deficient expression of adult hemoglobin. The genetically modified cells are then reinfused into the patient's circulation to take up residence in the bone marrow and thereby permit stable and prolonged expression of HbF from the patient's bone marrow. Whether this approach reaches the level of practical widespread clinical application remains to be seen.

*TALENs.* Bacterial virulence results from the introduction into infected cells of transcription activator-like effectors (TALEs) whose binding specificity to single base pairs in target cell DNA can be engineered to recognize and bind to lengthy sequences at any desired chromosomal locus. When fused with a catalytic domain such as Fok1, the complex is able to introduce double-stranded breaks at virtually any selected locus in a target chromosome. In 2014, Ramalingam and colleagues reported transcription activator-like effector nuclease (TALEN)-mediated site-specific correction of the mutations for cystic fibrosis, Gaucher's Disease and sickle cell anemia (10). In 2015, Waseem Qasim and the gene therapy team at Great Ormond Street Hospital in London took the technology to the bedside (11) and used a remarkable and complex combination of CAR-T and TALEN-mediated gene editing to treat an infant suffering from relapsed B-cell leukemia. They introduced the chimeric antigen receptor (CAR) for the B-cell antigen CD19 into universal donor T cells in which they also used a TALEN construct to knock out the resident T-cell receptor α chain and CD52 gene loci. The infant achieved a remarkable disease remission from this very complex first clinical application of TALEN editing for cancer immuno-gene therapy and showed only minimal short-term and self-limited adverse effects.

TALENs were quickly shown in preclinical in vitro studies to correct mutations for sickle cell anemia, Gaucher's disease, xeroderma pigmentosum and epidermolysis bullosum (12, 13). The TALEN editing system has been FDA approved for phase I clinical trials for hematological cancers such as acute myeloid leukemia, non-Hodgkin's lymphoma, multiple myeloma and cervical cancers, and in a Chinese phase I trial, to decrease the expression of human papilloma virus (HPV) E6/E7, to induce cell apoptosis and inhibit cell growth in cervical intraepithelial neoplasia. A trial sponsored by Allogene, Inc. combining a CD19-targeted CAR and an anti-CD52 TALEN is underway in patients with relapsed/refractory large B-cell lymphoma (LBCL). Although the results of this and similar studies have still to be reported, it seems likely that the TALEN approach to genome editing may find usefulness in some such combined CAR-T/TALEN editing scenarios. These kinds of editing protocols may very well be increasingly overshadowed by the next and the most important revolution of genome editing; i.e., CRISPR-Cas9 technology.

*CRISPR-Cas9 editing.* The CRISPR-Cas9 genome editing technology exploded onto the manipulative genetic scene after a short but intense history of studies of the acquired immune mechanisms that have evolved in bacteria and archaea to protect themselves from virus infection. As in the case of Zn-finger and TALEN editing, the underlying concept of the initial CRISPR-Cas9 editing strategies is the use of a targetable and programmable nuclease that binds to and produces double-strand cuts at a specific locus in the target DNA, allowing the host cell repair mechanisms of homology-directed repair (HDR) that sews over the scission or the non-homologous (NHEJ) repair mechanism that may lead to the introduction of short insertions or deletions (indels). Such events can knock out a target gene or insert an element with sequence homology to the target site.

CRISPR elements are a family of direct repeats in bacterial genomes that were described initially by Y. Ishino of Kyushu University in 1987 and Francis Mojica of the University of Alicante in Spain in 1993 (14, 15). It was Mojica who later coined the term CRISPR (clustered regularly interspaced short palindromic repeats). The CRISPR sequences were later found to be associated with adjacent families of scissors-like Cas endonucleases (CRISPR-associated proteins). Primary exposure of the prokaryote to a virus or other invading mobile genetic elements such as viruses or transposons leads to integration of short invader genome sequences into the CRISPR locus, thereby allowing the host organism to memorize the invader by expressing short invader-specific RNAs from the spacer-repeats which, during a secondary infection, interact with a Cas endonuclease and act as guides to the specific sequence in the invader genome and create double-stranded cuts in the invading genome at that site.

As arcane as this bit of prokaryotic genetics may seem, its versatility and power were recognized as the basis for a completely new approach to manipulative genetics that has brought about a revolution in virtually every aspect of biology, allowing creation of genetically modified animal and plant species, creation of vast new commercialization opportunities, and it has completely revolutionized experimental genetics. A complete description of the development of the CRISPR-Cas genome editing technology is far beyond the scope and capabilities of this book, but for the purpose of this historical view of gene therapy, it is not an exaggeration to state that the CRISPR-Cas genome editing system has created immensely powerful new approaches not only to human gene therapy but also genetic manipulations of all aspects of biomedicine and agriculture. As in all such all-encompassing scientific evolutions, the consequences are a mix of laudable and constructive effects and misguided and potentially dangerous and even unethical applications, as discussed in later chapters.

In 2012, several research groups more or less simultaneously adapted the CRISPR microbial adaptive immunity mechanisms, especially those found in *Streptococcus pyogenes*, *Staphylococcus aureus*, and *Streptococcus thermophilus*, to introduce targeted sequence edits into mammalian and other eucaryotic organisms. The CRISPR-Cas pioneering investigators included Virginius Sysknus in Latvia (16), Jennifer Doudna at the University of California in Berkeley (17) (Figure 19.1a), Emmanuelle Charpentier from the universities of Vienna and Umeå and the Max Planck Institute for Infection

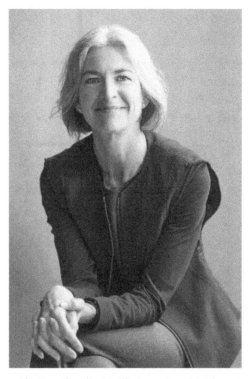

**Figure 19.1a.** Jennifer Doudna (b. 1964), American biochemistry and Shing Chancellor's Professor in Chemistry and cell biology at the University of California, Berkeley. She was principal developer of the CRISPR-Cas9 gene editing technology, and with her French colleague Emmanuelle Charpentier, she received the 2020 Nobel Prize for Chemistry. Courtesy of Innovative Genomics Institute, UC Berkeley.

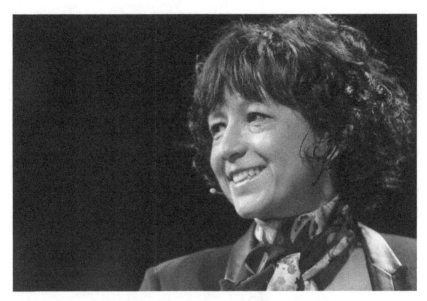

**Figure 19.1b.** Emmanuelle Charpentier (b. 1968), French microbiologist, geneticist and biochemist who shared the 2020 Nobel Prize in Chemistry. She serves as director at the Max Plank Institute for Infection Biology in Berlin. Reproduced with permission from Max Alexander, Science Photo Library.

Biology, Berlin (18) (Figure 19.2) and Feng Zhang at the Massachusetts (MIT) in Cambridge, Massachusetts (19). Doudna and Charpentier received the 2020 Nobel Prize in Chemistry, and Zhang, MIT and the Broad Institute were recognized by the award of the patent for their application of CRISPR-Cas9 editing techniques for genome editing in human cells, a crucial prerequisite for application to gene therapy.

The design of CRISPR-Cas9 genome editing is not a static technology, and improvements, modifications and extensions are being made at a furious pace. The goal of many of these changes is to reduce the incidence of unintended edits at unwanted sites in the genome (off-target effect), to specify more accurately in vivo the tissue target and to permit edits of multiple target genes, for instance, in a multigenic disorder.

For the powerful CRISPR-Cas-based gene editing technology to become most useful for the prevention and treatment of human genetic disease, it would be necessary to deliver the CRISPR-Cas9 complexes to human cells and tissues, especially in vivo, and to do so safely, efficiently and non-immunogenically. For that purpose, many of the well-established methods for gene transfer, including physical methods of electroporation, microinjection, and hydrodynamic injection, the use of nonviral systems such as lipid nanoparticles and adenovirus, lentivirus and AAV viral vectors are all being adapted to the in vitro and in vivo delivery of CRISPR-Cas editing complexes.

*CRISPR clinical trials—China, United States, Europe.* The explosive announcement in 2012 of successful genome editing by CRISPR-Cas9 technology set off a furious international race to human clinical application. The idea of clinically useful genome editing was not novel to the CRISPR-Cas9 system, since the zinc finger and TALEN editing tools had already been used successfully to knock out CCR5 and CXCR4 receptors to prevent HIV infection and in multiple clinical trials of hematological malignancies, and of course a number of Mendelian genetic diseases such as factor IX hemophilia B, mucopolysaccharidosis types I and II and others. But the ease of construction and use of CRISPR-Cas9 tools and the promising, but the somewhat slower clinical progress with alternative editing approaches catalyzed the application of CRISPR-Cas9 editing to a human clinical trial. Clinical therapeutic targets have included genome editing, base editing, gene regulation and gene activation (20).

By 2024, a wide variety of common and rare diseases have become targets for CRISPR editing clinical trials, and have included blood disorders such as hemophilias and sickle cell disease, cancers, genetic blindness, chronic infections, muscular dystrophies and rare genetic disorders. In 2016 a mere 4 years after the 2012 announcement of the CRISPR-Cas9 genome editing methods, the Chinese investigators You Lu and Tony Mok in Hong Kong undertook a phase I clinical trial of CRISPR–Cas9 *PD-1*-edited T cells in patients with advanced non-small-cell lung cancer (21). They showed that the use of such cells in humans is safe, and recognizing the limitations of such early-stage technology, they cautioned wisely that "future trials should use superior gene editing approaches to improve therapeutic efficacy."

The first CRISPR-based clinical study in the United States was a complex 2020 phase I triple-target genome editing study in autologous T cells from three patients with myeloma and metastatic bone sarcoma (22). Two T cell receptor (TCR) chains, TCRα (*TRAC*) and TCRβ (*TRBC*), were deleted to allow expression of a synthetic, cancer T cell receptor transgene (NY-ESO-1). In addition, the gene encoding the programmed cell death protein 1 (PD-1; *PDCD1*), was deleted. The modified T cells engrafted and persisted for 9 months, further proving that the combined CAR-T/CRISPR-Cas9 editing approach was safe and had great promise in immunotherapy for at least some forms of cancer.

During the same time, many CRISPR-based genomic editing trials were reported from a growing list of biotech and pharma firms. One of the first and most influential came from the genome editing biotech firm Editas Medicine, a Cambridge, Massachusetts, biotech firm and one of the leaders in clinical CRISPR editing. This early clinical trial was for the progressive blindness disorder Leber's congenital amaurosis (LCA), the same disorder treated more than a decade earlier by Bennett and her colleagues at Penn using a "traditional" gene therapy approach of AAV virus–mediated gene transfer. The CRISPR-mediated genome editing clinical trial involves subretinal injection of a CRISPR-Cas9 complex containing a guide RNA designed to remove the mutation in the responsible CEP290 gene, restore normal mRNA and protein expression and restore some useful visual acuity. Gratifyingly, 3 of the 14 treated patients showed improvement in vision, but Editas chose to concentrate on other clinical CRISPR editing applications such as sickle cell anemia and halted the Leber's study.

In both the United States and Europe, a CRISPR-editing approach to correct the severe anemia in both sickle cell disease and beta-thalassemia has involved restoration of expression of fetal hemoglobin rather than correction of the underlying sickle cell or thalassemia mutations. The common approach in several of these phase I human clinical trials has been to induce expression of fetal hemoglobin (HbF) to take the place of the deficient expression of adult hemoglobin A. In 2022, Editas reported encouraging safety and efficacy results in several patients suffering from severe sickle cell disease using this CRISPR editing approach. The study involved the use of a variant of endonuclease AsCas12a rather than Cas9 to edit the promoter regions of gamma globin genes 1 and 2 to restore HbF production and thereby recapitulate the natural mechanism of fetal hemoglobin persistence to replace the deficient hemoglobin production in sickle cell disease. Treated patients showed markedly improved total hemoglobin blood levels and had no clinically significant vaso-occlusive events for prolonged periods after many months.

The pioneering biotech firm CRISPR Therapeutics/Vertex in Cambridge, Massachusetts, has also developed a similar CRISPR-based editing products for sickle cell disease and beta-thalassemia. An alternative phase I clinical trial pursued by bluebird bio to treat sickle cell disease by transducing hematopoietic stem cells (HSPCs) transduced with the BB305 lentiviral vector encoding an anti-sickling globin gene with an amino acid substitution (threonine to glutamine at position 87) that sterically inhibits polymerization of sickle hemoglobin. In Europe, bluebird bio obtained the first EMA approval for a gene therapy for transfusion-dependent thalassemia (TDT) using the same lentivirus-mediated approach, LentiGlobin (Zynteglo) (betibeglogene autotemcel), as applied in its clinical trial for sickle cell disease. In 2021, German regulators denied European sale of Zynteglo because of the $1.8 million asking price for Zynteglo in the European market. On the other hand, at the present time, Zynteglo is still approved in the United States for use in patients suffering from beta-thalassemia and soon to be approved for sickle cell disease.

In 2021, scientists at the biotech firms Vertex and CRISPR Therapeutics reported a HbF induction strategy similar to that developed by *bluebird bio* that used the editing product CTX001 in hematopoietic stem cells to target the transcription factor BCL11A that represses γ-globin expression and fetal hemoglobin production. Several thalassemia and sickle cell anemia patients showed increased levels of fetal hemoglobin and transfusion-independence and reduced vaso-occlusive events. Rather than attempting to correct the sickle cell mutation responsible for production of mutant HbS, these gene editing trials for sickle cell anemia have preferred to induce the expression of gamma globin and the resulting production of fetal hemoglobin that physiologically treats the anemia. But, of course, in the long run, the sequence-correction editing attack directly on the HbS mutation itself is inevitable and eventually is likely to become the preferred treatment of choice for sickle cell anemia. The recent development of base editing technology makes such a direct attack and sequence correction of disease-related genes inevitable and preferable. Sickle cell disease will almost certainly be one of the very first common genetic diseases to be treated by CRISPR-mediated genome editing.

Many additional CRISPR editing clinical trials will come quickly in the near future and have already begun to appear for both a variety of rare as well as common diseases. In 2019, the FDA approved CRISPR-based therapy for life-threatening transthyretin amyloidosis (also called ATTR amyloidosis) in which CRISPR editing has reduced accumulation of the toxic TTR protein in neural and cardiac tissue. Muscular dystrophy is an obvious and appealing target disease crying out for gene editing therapeutic approaches. One CRISPR-Cas9-based study carried out by Cure Rare Disease (CRD) and intended to induce expression of an alternate form of the dystrophin protein was complicated by the death of the single patient, although the roles of the gene editing procedure, if any, and possible cardiac toxicity of the AAV delivery vector have not been firmly established. Equally stunning has been the demonstration in 2024 by Intellia Therapeutics in Cambridge that CRISPR-based therapy results in >95% reduction of severe angioedema attacks in patients with hereditary angioedema.

In addition to Mendelian genetic disease, some forms of infectious diseases have also come under attack by CRISPR-based editing strategies. LocusBiosciences of Research Triangle Park in North Carolina has reported good results with therapy for urinary tract infection, using CRISPR-Cas3-edited bacteriophage that is targeted by CRISPR-Ca3 editing to destroy infecting bacterial in urinary tract infections after direct bladder instillation. Although previous studies have shown that zinc finger knockout of HIV receptors CCR5 and CXCR4 in human holds promise for prevention and treatment of HIV infection, similar studies with CRISPR-Cas9 editing have not yet reached the clinical trial stage of treatment for established HIV-1 infections. But they will certainly come.

And come they have! With stunning speed, several iterations of now "traditional" CRISPR-Cas9 genome editing techniques have made such advances a reality. They have made possible some answers to the next obvious questions regarding genome editing—1) if the target genetic defect is simply a single base pair mutation, would it be possible simply to correct one base to restore a normal wild-type genomic sequence and thereby correct a disease-causing point mutation, and 2) would it be possible to insert entire therapeutic sequences or delete or substitute unwanted sequences without having to create double-strand breaks in the target genome? The answer to both questions is "yes," as proven first through the pioneering work of David Liu and colleagues at Harvard University in both cases as well as other geneticists through the development of "base editing" and "prime editing." Both of these techniques take advantage of the use of catalytically inactive forms of Cas9 to create nicks rather than double-strand breaks in the target genome.

***Base editing.*** Base editing (24) takes advantage of the use of the catalytically inactive Cas9 fused with a base-modifying enzyme like adenine deaminase or cytidine deaminase that serves to chemically modify a target nucleotide. Modified and catalytically "dead" CRISPR-Cas tools bring about single-base edits because their disabled nuclease domains can produce only nicks rather than double-strand breaks in the target DNA. When coupled with base-modifying enzymes such as adenine or cytidine deaminase, the Cas variants produce chemical changes at single base sites in the DNA through deamination of adenosine to inosine or cytidine to uridine, changes that are then resolved as guanosine or thymidine, resulting in C:G to A:T interconversions. Further developments of base-editing technology coupled with safe and efficient delivery mechanisms will eventually find a place in correction of disease-related point mutations by methods that will grow from these early base-editing tools. Additional CRISPR-based applications have been developed to edit processes that drive regulation and gene activation and suppression through epigenetic mechanisms of DNA methylation and histone acetylation. Amazingly, the use of zinc finger techniques for base editing of mitochondrial DNA have also been developed (23). It is extremely early days for these technologies to emerge and develop.

*Prime editing.* A next startling iteration of the genome editing revolution has come in the form of "prime editing," developed by Liu and colleagues (24, 25). The approach involves the use of an inactive Cas9 fused to a modified reverse transcriptase and a prime-editing guide RNA (pegRNA) that searches out the target site in the DNA genome and that provides the sequences that serve to replace the target DNA sequences and thereby create a correcting insertion, deletion, exon replacement or exon skipping or other genetic changes. The power of prime editing together with the precision of its effects ensures that it will become the approach of choice for many genome editing applications. To underscore that promise, the biotech company Prime Medicine received in 2024 FDA approval to begin a clinical trial for the immunodeficiency chronic granulomatous disease (CGD).

## References

1. Smithies O, Gregg RG, Boggs SS, Koralewski MA, Kucherlapati RS. Insertion of DNA sequences into the human chromosomal beta-globin locus by homologous recombination. *Nature.* 1985;317(6034):230–234.
2. Thomas KR, Folger KR, Capecchi MR. High frequency targeting of genes to specific sites in the mammalian genome. *Cell.* 1986;44:419–428.
3. Mansour SL, Thomas KR, Capecchi MR. Disruption of the proto-oncogene int-2 in mouse embryo-derived stem cells: a general strategy for targeting mutations to non-selectable genes. *Nature.* 1988;336:348–352.
4. Klug A. The discovery of zinc fingers and their development for practical applications in gene regulation and genome manipulation. *Q Rev Biophys.* 2010 Feb;43(1):1–21. doi: 10.1017/S0033583510000089. Epub 2010 May 18. PMID: 20478078 Review.
5. Rebar EJ, Pabo CO. Zinc finger phage: affinity selection of fingers with new DNA-binding specificities. *Science.* 1994 Feb 4;263(5147):671–673. doi: 10.1126/science.8303274. PMID: 8303274.

6. Ramalingam S, Annaluru N, Kandavelou K, Chandrasegaran S. TALEN-mediated generation and genetic correction of disease-specific human induced pluripotent stem cells. *Current Gene Therapy.* 2014;14(6):461–472. doi:10.2174/1566523214666140918101725. PMID: 25245091.
7. Urnov FD, Rebar EJ, Holmes MC, Zhang HS, Gregory PD. Genome editing with engineered zinc finger nucleases. *Nat Rev Genet.* 2010 Sep;11(9):636–646. doi: 10.1038/nrg2842.PMID: 20717154 Review.
8. Tebas P, Stein D, Tang WW, Frank I, Wang SQ, Lee G, et al. Gene editing of CCR5 in autologous CD4 T cells of persons infected with HIV. *N Engl J Med.* 2014;370(10):901–910.
9. Didigu CA, Wilen CB, Wang J, Duong J, Secreto AJ, Danet-Desnoyers GA, Riley JL, Gregory PD, June CH, Holmes MC, Doms RW. Simultaneous zinc-finger nuclease editing of the HIV coreceptors ccr5 and cxcr4 protects CD4+ T cells from HIV-1 infection. *Blood.* 2014 Jan 2;123(1):61–69. doi: 10.1182/blood-2013-08-521229. Epub 2013 Oct 25. PMID: 24162716.
10. Ramalingam S, Annaluru N, Kandavelou K, Chandrasegaran S. TALEN-mediated generation and genetic correction of disease-specific human induced pluripotent stem cells. *Curr Gene Ther.* 2014;14(6):461–472. doi: 10.2174/1566523214666140918101725. PMID: 25245091.
11. Qasim W, Amrolia PJ, Samarasinghe S, et al. First clinical application of Talen engineered universal CAR19 T cells in B-ALL. *Blood.* 2015;126:2046.
12. Dupuy A, Valton J, Leduc S, Armier J, Galetto R, Gouble A, Lebuhotel C, Stary A, Pâques F, Duchateau P, Sarasin A, Daboussi F. Targeted gene therapy of xeroderma pigmentosum cells using meganuclease and TALEN™. *PLOS ONE.* 2013;8(11):e78678. Bibcode:2013PLoSO...878678D. doi: 10.1371/journal.pone.0078678. PMC 3827243. PMID: 24236034.
13. Osborn MJ, Starker CG, McElroy AN, Webber BR, Riddle MJ, Xia L, DeFeo AP, Gabriel R, Schmidt M, von Kalle C, Carlson DF, Maeder ML, Joung JK, Wagner JE, Voytas DF, Blazar BR, Tolar J. TALEN-based gene correction for epidermolysis bullosa. *Mol Ther.* 2013 June;21(6):1151–1159. doi: 10.1038/mt.2013.56. PMC 3677309. PMID: 23546300.
14. Ishino Y, Shinagawa H, Makino K, Amemura M, Nakata A. Nucleotide sequence of the iap gene, responsible for alkaline phosphatase isozyme conversion in Escherichia coli, and identification of the gene product. *J Bacteriol.* 1987 Dec;169(12):5429–5433. doi: 10.1128/jb.169.12.5429-5433.1987. PMID: 3316184.
15. Mojica FJ, Juez G, Rodríguez-Valera F. Transcription at different salinities of Haloferax mediterranei sequences adjacent to partially modified PstI sites. *Mol Microbiol.* 1993 Aug;9(3):613–621. doi: 10.1111/j.1365-2958.1993.tb01721.x. PMID: 8412707.
16. Gasiunas G, Barrangou R, Horvath P, Siksnys V. Cas9-crRNA ribonucleoprotein complex mediates specific DNA cleavage for adaptive immunity in bacteria. *Proc Natl Acad Sci U S A.* 2012 Sep 25;109(39):E2579– E2586. doi: 10.1073/pnas.1208507109. Epub 2012 Sep 4.
17. Jinek M, Chylinski K, Fonfara I, Hauer M, Doudna JA, Charpentier E. A programmable dual-RNA-guided DNA endonuclease in adaptive bacterial immunity. *Science.* 2012 Aug 17;337(6096):816–821. doi: 10.1126/science.1225829. Epub 2012 Jun 28. PMID: 22745249 Free PMC article.
18. Wiedenheft B, Sternberg SH, Doudna JA. RNA-guided genetic silencing systems in bacteria and archaea. *Nature.* 2012 Feb 15;482(7385):331–338. doi: 10.1038/nature10886. PMID: 22337052 Review.
19. Zhang J, Rouillon C, Kerou M, Reeks J, Brugger K, Graham S, Reimann J, Cannone G, Liu H, Albers SV, Naismith JH, Spagnolo L, White MF. Structure and mechanism of the CMR complex for CRISPR-mediated antiviral immunity. *Mol Cell.* 2012 Feb 10;45(3):303–313. doi: 10.1016/j.molcel.2011.12.013. Epub 2012 Jan 5. PMID: 22227115.
20. Doudna JA. The promise and challenge of therapeutic genome editing. *Nature.* 2020 Feb;578(7794):229–236. doi: 10.1038/s41586-020-1978-5. Epub 2020 Feb 12. PMID: 32051598.

21. Lu Y, Xue J, Deng T, Zhou X, Yu K, Deng L, Huang M, Yi X, Liang M, Wang Y, Shen H, Tong R, Wang W, Li L, Song J, Li J, Su X, Ding Z, Gong Y, Zhu J, Wang Y, Zou B, Zhang Y, Li Y, Zhou L, Liu Y, Yu M, Wang Y, Zhang X, Yin L, Xia X, Zeng Y, Zhou Q, Ying B, Chen C, Wei Y, Li W, Mok T. Safety and feasibility of CRISPR-edited T cells in patients with refractory non-small-cell lung cancer. *Nat Med*. 2020 May;26(5):732–740. doi: 10.1038/s41591-020-0840-5. Epub 2020 Apr 27. PMID: 32341578.
22. Stadtmauer EA, Fraietta JA, Davis MM, Cohen AD, Weber KL, Lancaster E, Mangan PA, Kulikovskaya I, Gupta M, Chen F, Tian L, Gonzalez VE, Xu J, Jung IY, Melenhorst JJ, Plesa G, Shea J, Matlawski T, Cervini A, Gaymon AL, Desjardins S, Lamontagne A, Salas-Mckee J, Fesnak A, Siegel DL, Levine BL, Jadlowsky JK, Young RM, Chew A, Hwang WT, Hexner EO, Carreno BM, Nobles CL, Bushman FD, Parker KR, Qi Y, Satpathy AT, Chang HY, Zhao Y, Lacey SF, June CH. CRISPR-engineered T cells in patients with refractory cancer. *Science*. 2020 Feb 28;367(6481):eaba7365. doi: 10.1126/science.aba7365. Epub 2020 Feb 6. PMID: 32029687.
23. Willis JCW, Silva-Pinheiro P, Widdup L, Minczuk M, Liu DR. Compact zinc finger base editors that edit mitochondrial or nuclear DNA in vitro and in vivo. *Nat Commun*. 2022 Nov 23;13(1):7204. doi: 10.1038/s41467-022-34784-7. PMID: 36418298.
24. Komor AC, Kim YB, Packer MS, Zuris JA, Liu DR. Programmable editing of a target base in genomic DNA without double-stranded DNA cleavage. *Nature*. 2016 May 19;533(7603):420–424.
25. Anzalone AV, Randolph PB, Davis JR, Sousa AA, Koblan LW, Levy JM, Chen PJ, Wilson C, Newby GA, Raguram A, Liu DR. Search-and-replace genome editing without double-strand breaks or donor DNA. *Nature*. 2019 Dec;576(7785):149–157. doi: 10.1038/s41586-019-1711-4. Epub 2019 Oct 21.

# 20
# RNA-based therapies and programmable RNA editing

DNA-based clustered, prime editing interspaced short palindromic repeats (CRISPR)-modulated genome editing has completely and irrevocably transformed the concept of disease and therapy. But DNA is not the only actor in that drama, and other cellular processes and components likely play important and still undefined roles in health and disease. RNA-based therapies are surely going to become a dominant form of gene therapy by targeting the several attractive functions that RNA plays in pathogenesis of normal and pathogenic cellular functions. Classically, most approaches to gene-based therapies have emphasized an attack on the aberrant structure and pathogenic function of DNA as the ultimate repository of all genetic information. It is through DNA that we have come to understand how mutations lead to the biochemical and metabolic functions that underlie most human disease. It is therefore no surprise that attempts to develop genetic therapies have focused largely on DNA and its content and expression of genes. But there is much more to human disease and to therapy than merely manipulating DNA. The business end of gene expression lies in the various classes of RNA that convert encoded genetic information into physiological functions, and therefore a number of alternative and very promising pathways to therapy have emerged based on tools that target and modify specific gene expression though these RNA intermediaries.

*RNA editing tools and targets.* Some of the most widely used prototype RNA-modulating agents have been single-stranded antisense synthetic oligonucleotides (ASOs) such as small interfering RNAs (siRNAs). There are a number of attractive tools and targets for RNA-based therapeutics that generally are designed to degrade or interfere with the role of messenger RNAs (mRNAs), the role of small double-stranded interfering RNAs (siRNAs) in cleaving and degrading specific target mRNAs, the functions of short hairpin RNAs (shRNAs) that are stably and readily introduced by viral vectors into mammalian cells, the role of antisense single-stranded oligonucleotides

(ASOs) that recognize and bind to specific mRNA sequences and render the resulting duplexes susceptible to degradation by RNase H, or the function of single-stranded oligonucleotides that bind to diverse classes of proteins and interfere with their functionally required protein–protein interactions. These approaches to RNA-based therapy are straightforward logical applications of known RNA function and reasonable candidates for therapeutic use.

Among the currently most well-known of the RNA-based therapies are nusinersen (Spinraza), an antisense oligo (ASO) nucleotide approved by the Food and Drug Administration (FDA) in 2016 to treat spinal muscular atrophy, and a variety of aptamer treatments for forms of retinal disease. Nusinersen represents a breakthrough milestone approach to gene-based therapy of the fatal degenerative neurological disease spinomuscular atrophy (SMA). It is essentially a splice-altering oligonucleotide that restores expression of the survival motor neuron protein (SMN) by increasing the splicing efficiency of the SMN2 pre-mRNA and thereby serves to prevent neuron degeneration that results from SMN deficiency. The ASO nusinersen was the astounding first effective treatment for this utterly devastating childhood neurodegenerative disease, but the requirement for repeated intrathecal administration spurred the search for alternative gene-based therapies. As with other ASOs, nusinersen has the disadvantage of not being suitable for vector-based delivery and thereby for becoming encoded in target DNA. These ASOs must therefore be delivered chronically during the entire duration of therapy. A more permanent and durable form of therapy for SMA emerged with the development and 2019 FDA approval of the adeno-associated virus (AAV)-based gene transfer of the vector Zolgesma that expresses a functional copy of a wild-type SMN1 gene (1). This therapeutic approach was consistent with much of the thinking at the time of virus-vector, especially AAV, mediated gene transfer. In contrast to the need for continuous treatment with the ASO agent nusinersen to prevent neurodegeneration and early neuronal death in SMA, the AAV-mediated reconstitution of neuronal function by Zolgesma represents a stable and one-time administration that makes it, at least at the present time, the current treatment of choice for this intractable and lethal neurodegenerative disease.

In addition to SMA, ASO oligonucleotide-based therapy has gained great attraction for additional degenerative neurological diseases, including amyotrophic lateral sclerosis (ALS) or frontotemporal dementia (FTD). In 2023, the FDA approved a Phase III trial of the antisense oligonucleotide Qalsody (tofersen) in patients with the form of ALS caused by mutations in the superoxide dismutase (SOD1) gene. Qalsody is an antisense oligonucleotide that targets SOD1 mRNA to reduce the synthesis of SOD1 protein.

In addition, the biotech firm WAVE received approval in 2021 for a trial of their antisense oligonucleotide WVE-004 that targets mutations in the gene C9ORF72 that causes amyotrophic lateral sclerosis and frontotemporal dementia by producing hexanucleotide repeats in the C9ORF72 mRNA that is expressed in a neurotoxic dipeptide protein gene product. The WAVE ASO mediates degradation of hexanucleotide expansion-containing C9ORF72 mRNA, and its safety following intrathecal administration is being tested in a multicenter phase 1 trial in patients with ALS and FTD.

Unlike ASOs, siRNA oligos can be delivered in vivo by viral vectors such as AAV, but such approaches can be complicated by the immunogenicity of double-stranded RNA and unwanted off-target effects.

The first FDA-approved aptamer-based clinical trial for eye disease, Macugen, was FDA approved in 2004 and was targeted against vascular endothelial growth factor (VEGF) to inhibit the neovascularization associated with wet macular degeneration. Following the removal of Macugen from the market, additional VEGF inhibitors such as the Genentech product Lucentis and Eylea from Regeneron have become treatments of choice for wet macular degeneration, diabetic retinopathy and additional retinal diseases. The importance of these breakthrough treatments is attested by their combined sales on $8 billion in 2021. They are revolutionizing the treatment of severe debilitating eye disease.

*Programmable RNA-based RNA editing.* While the CRISPR-Cas9 gene editing technology has opened vast new areas for genetic research and for gene-based therapy, there are situations where it might not be ideal to create permanent changes in the genome, or where it might be desirable to make genetic changes reversible. Under such conditions, it would be preferable to target the RNA end of the central dogma of genetic information flow by specifically editing the structure, regulation and expression of RNAs and RNA effector proteins. The extension of the firmly established and even "classical" CRISPR-Cas editing tools to RNA editing targeting is now emerging and evolving very quickly. Recently, the concepts and tools of CRISPR-Cas9-based genome editing with its potential for directly affecting RNA functions have been applied in stunning fashion to make RNA a direct target for genetic manipulation rather than merely a consequence of DNA editing (2, 3). This advance has involved discovery of a variety of other Cas13 and Cas12 proteins that target RNA instead of DNA as does Cas9, tools that have led to the astounding capabilities of editing at the level of single bases ("base editing") (4) and to powerful and effective methods to replace entire long sequence elements ("prime editing") (5). These new Cas13 techniques have led to programmable manipulation of splicing mechanisms allowing A-to-I (RNA editing for programmable adenosine replacement—"REPAIR"), RNA editing for specific C-to-U exchange ("RESCUE") and C-to-U RNA editor ("CURE") editing. Possibly even more important for many genetic diseases is a technology called "prime editing" that not only can carry out base editing but also can direct the removal or insertion of kilobase DNA sequences into the genome.

These amazing new technologies will almost certainly constitute the basis for much of gene therapy in the future.

### References

1. Mendell JR, Al-Zaidy S, Shell R, Arnold WD, Rodino-Klapac LR, Prior TW, Lowes L, Alfano L, Berry K, Church K, Kissel JT, Nagendran S, L'Italien J, Sproule DM, Wells C, Cardenas JA, Heitzer MD, Kaspar A, Corcoran S, Braun L, Likhite S, Miranda C, Meyer K, Foust KD, Burghes AHM, Kaspar BK. Single-dose gene-replacement therapy for spinal muscular atrophy. *N Engl J Med.* 2017 Nov 2;377(18):1713–1722. doi: 10.1056/NEJMoa1706198.
2. Abudayyeh OO, Gootenberg JS, Essletzbichler P, Han S, Joung J, Belanto JJ, Verdine V, Cox DBT, Kellner MJ, Regev A, Lander ES, Voytas DF, Ting AY, Zhang F. RNA targeting with CRISPR-Cas13. *Nature.* 2017 Oct 12;550(7675):280–284. doi: 10.1038/nature24049. Epub 2017 Oct 4.
3. Qian Y, Li J, Zhao S, et al. Programmable RNA sensing for cell monitoring and manipulation. *Nature.* 2022;610:713–721. https://doi.org/10.1038/s41586-022-05280-1.
4. Huang TP, Newby GA, Liu DR. Precision genome editing using cytosine and adenine base editors in mammalian cells. *Nat Protoc.* 2021 Feb;16(2):1089–1128. doi: 10.1038/s41596-020-00450-9. Epub 2021 Jan 18.
5. Anzalone AV, Koblan LW, Liu DR. Genome editing with CRISPR-Cas nucleases, base editors, transposases and prime editors. *Nat Biotechnol.* 2020 Jul;38(7):824–844. doi: 10.1038/s41587-020-0561-9. Epub 2020 Jun 22.

# 21

# The role of biotech and pharma in the development of gene therapy

With the remarkable and largely academically driven genetic augmentation successes with both the adenosine deaminase (ADA)-deficiency and X-linked forms of severe combined immunodeficiency disease (SCID) and the encouraging and at least partial clinical success in patients suffering from Leber's congenital amaurosis blindness, the field of gene therapy took major steps away from its deeply discouraging era to one of optimism, to broadly optimistic anticipation and acceptance by the biomedical and general public communities and to rapidly expanding scientific and funding support from the biotech and pharmaceutical firms. By the first decades of the 21st century, technical and preclinical progress gained speed to the point where hundreds of gene therapy studies were being carried out and were producing proof-of-concept results in many human disease models. Although academia was the major force in the early conceptual development of gene therapy, the production of clinical-grade gene transfer reagents and vectors and the development and implementation of clinical trials were rapidly becoming dependent on far greater resources that would be available only from biotech, big pharma and, to a limited extent, philanthropy. Academia itself does not have the interest, the experience or the financial or logistical resources to bring new therapies to clinical reality. For that reason, the explosive growth of biotech and big pharma was a vital catalyst in the maturation of the field of gene therapy during the latter parts of the 20th century and the early decades of the 21st century, especially in the United States and Europe.

Much of the early development of gene-based biotech took place in California. One of the first and most well-known start-up biotech firms was Cetus Corp., founded in Berkeley, California in 1971. Initially, interests at Cetus were not directly in questions of gene therapy but rather in improved production of antibiotics and vaccines, but with the advent of the recombinant DNA technology, Cetus undertook the cloning and production of interferon for possible cancer therapy purposes. But Cetus became far more recognized as the home for the development by Karry Mullis of polymerase chain reaction (PCR) for analytic and production applications of DNA, almost certainly the most important central core technology in virtually all of modern genetic science (1). Mullis received the 1993 Nobel Prize in Physiology or Medicine.

But the giant in the nascent genetics biotechnology world in the United States was a new start-up biotech firm in San Francisco called Genentech, Inc., founded in 1976 in San Francisco by Herbert Boyer and the venture capitalist Robert Swanson of the San Francisco venture capital firm Kleiner, Perkins, Caufield and Byers. The goal of Genentech was to deliver on the promise of the recombinant DNA revolution that was taking place at the time by creating an entirely new approach to gene-based therapeutics. Genentech quickly delivered on that promise. Because Genentech had no laboratory facilities of its own, Boyer and Swanson collaborated with Keiichi Itakura and Arthur Riggs at nearby City of Hope first, as a proof of principle, to clone and produce the hormone somatostatin (1). But at Swanson's urging, the ultimate goal of the Genentech team was to produce a commercially valuable product and get it to the market and to patients. Even though there were two obvious candidates for that role (i.e., human growth hormone for treating dwarfism and human insulin for treating diabetes), the true long-term holy grail was insulin.

At that time, insulin was obtained by the awkward and expensive method of isolating it from cow and pig pancreas, a process that required the retrieval of glands from more than 20,000 animals and that could yield only enough insulin to treat a few hundred human diabetic patients, hardly a dent in the world need for insulin. A method to use recombinant tools to produce active insulin would be an enormous advance and would benefit millions of diabetic patients worldwide! Very quickly, the combined Genentech and City of Hope groups reproduced the methods that they used to clone and produce somatostatin to produce both polypeptide chains of human insulin, which they combined in transfected *E. coli* to produce biologically active single-chain insulin. The resulting technology was licensed to the Indianapolis pharma Eli Lilly Inc., and in 1982, the resulting synthetic insulin, marketed as Humulin, was approved by the Food and Drug Administration (FDA) for human use. It was an immense scientific and commercial triumph! Almost simultaneously, the Genentech team used similar recombinant DNA methods to produce synthetic recombinant human growth hormone, which was approved by the FDA in 1985 and which joined insulin as the first recombinant products to reach the market. These triumphs by Genentech and the City of Hope scientists demonstrated that recombinant DNA methods could produce biologically active protein gene products and could therefore play a role in the treatment of genetic disease by the principles of metabolite replacement concept implied in Garrod's concept of "inborn errors of metabolism." Recombinant DNA technology was certainly about to deliver therapies for genetic disease, but these advances were still only improved drug developments—still not quite "gene therapy."

Other new biotech companies were developing additional applications of the tools and concepts of recombinant DNA technology and growing understanding of molecular and cellular biology and the potential for gene-based therapies. Many of these early companies emerged as spin-offs in the academic scientific centers, most notably in Boston, San Francisco and San Diego. Such companies included Biogen, the Swiss-American company devoted to applying the DNA sequencing technology developed by one of the company's founders Walter Gilbert to biomedical problems, initially for diagnostics and vaccine development for hepatitis B. Biogen's activities in the field of gene therapy were to come later in the beginning of the 21st century.

Among the first and most influential of the San Diego companies was Hybridtech Inc. founded in 1978 by the UCSD cancer physician Ivor Royston and entrepreneur Howard Birndorf for the purpose of developing cancer therapies based on the use of monoclonal antibody tools. Encouraged by the success of Hybridtech at attracting venture capital private sector financial support, a number of other physicians at UCSD in La Jolla founded Vical Inc., more directly interested in developing gene therapy tools and techniques. Vical recruited Phil Felgner from Syntex in Palo Alto who went on to develop the use of cationic lipids to introduce DNA and RNA into human and other eukaryotic cells, a core technology in much of modern gene therapy research.

As the tempo of academic gene therapy increased beginning in the early 1990s, it became increasingly evident that the technical and logistical know-how, deep financial pockets and resources of biotechnology and pharmaceutical firms would be required to take the field successfully to the clinic. One of the earliest of the gene therapy biotech firms was the very influential French biotech firm Genethon, established in 1990 by the French Muscular Dystrophy Association and the French muscular dystrophy charity Telethon. Genethon was devoted initially to the broad area of human genetics and the

Human Genome Project, and in 1993 the company switched its emphasis to gene therapy.

An additional influential gene therapy biotech company was Genetic Therapy Inc. (GTI) founded in Gaithersburg, Maryland, by French Anderson for the purpose of producing the retrovirus vector for the National Institutes of Health–based clinical trial of ADA-SCID. GTI served as the springboard for Anderson's 1992 clinical trial of ADA-SCID gene therapy but did not make major conceptual or technical advances and failed to survive.

As these and other start-up biotechs were establishing themselves in studies increasingly centered around gene therapy, most major pharmaceutical firms took only fleeting interest in gene therapy. The advent of one-time definitive gene-based treatments for illnesses, especially for the rare diseases as first envisioned for gene therapy, was inconsistent with corporate profit-based business models and were less attractive than long-term drug-based therapies even in genetic diseases as was the case for chronic diseases such as cancer and cardiovascular disease. But as biotech-driven gene therapy technology matured and became more credible and revealed not only the need for extensive production facilities and for large-scale clinical infrastructure but also enormous commercial and marketing opportunities, interest by big pharma grew and quickly became the principal driving force in delivering gene therapy studies and products to the public. In the period from 2000 to the present time of early 2020s, basic preclinical academic advances and early-stage clinical trials led to the emergence of many collaborations between the academic and private sector communities in the form of financial backing from pharmaceutical and biotechnology firms for academic research programs, for vector production and manufacturing and for support of clinical trials. Those collaborations have become one of the mainstays of cell and gene therapy.

The first approved and commercially licensed gene therapy in the Western world was the adenovirus vector-based gene therapy agent *Glybera* developed by Amsterdam Molecular Therapeutics (AMT) and the biotech firm uniQure and was approved by the European Medicine Agency in 2012 for the treatment of the extremely rare disorder of lipid metabolism and pancreatic and cardiovascular function caused by deficiency of the enzyme lipoprotein lipase. One of the several problems with this proposed treatment was the fact that it came on the market with a price of approximately one million dollars, taking it out of reach of patients and insurance payers. Furthermore, there were simply too few eligible patients to make the therapy commercially feasible and, together with the failure to secure FDA approval in the United States, *Glybera* was withdrawn in 2017. The failure of *Glybera* introduced the new complication of commercially supported gene therapies that came with virtually all subsequent gene therapy "successes" to the present day—their extremely high costs of up to several millions of dollars to patients. Individual patients and insurance carriers will not be willing or able to endure such costs as the field of gene therapy faces the formidable and politically sensitive task of bringing the technology to the bedside at reasonable costs to patients and to insurance carriers.

Following the commercial and logistical failure of *Glybera*, the maturing gene therapy technology, especially the use of AAV (adeno-associated virus) vectors, and expanding support from industry led to a series of more successful clinical applications. These advances have included effective commercially supported and licensed one-time therapies approved by both the U.S. FDA and the European Medicines Agency (EMA) for a number of genetic diseases, including RPE65 Leber's congenital amaurosis, using an AAV vector (*Luxturna*, Spark Therapeutics Inc.), spinal muscular atrophy (SMA), using an AAV vector (*Zolgensma*, Novartis Gene Therapies, Inc.), hemophilia A, using an AAV vector (*Rocktavian*, BioMarin, Inc.), hemophilia B, using an AAV vector (*Hemgenix*, CSL Behring).

Some of the early big pharma involvements in the field of gene therapy took the form of research and clinical support and alliances with academic gene therapy centers such as the influential and trend-setting $27 million 2012 Novartis–University of Pennsylvania alliance for cell and gene therapy and CAR-T programs, the broad Glaxo-SmithKline–Telethon gene therapy program at the San Rafaele Hospital in Milan funded with an initial infusion of $13 million. Those early efforts are becoming less and less impressive in light of the more recent parade of head-spinning mergers and acquisitions involving giant pharma firms such as Pfizer, Roche, Novartis, Biogen, UniQure, Spark Therapeutics, Sangamo Therapeutics, which amount to an industry-wide gene therapy valuation estimate of a market of $18 billion in 2022 and a projected market valuation of $94 billion by 2030. Recent examples of such pharma-biotech-academia ventures include the 2016 Biogen–Penn $2 billion alliance for ocular, muscle and central nervous system (CNS) gene therapy, the $3 billion alliance between WAVE Life Inc. of Cambridge, Massachusetts, and Takeda Pharmaceuticals for siRNA- and other RNA-based therapies for CNS diseases such as Huntington's disease, amyotrophic lateral sclerosis (ALS), frontotemporal dementia, and spinocerebellar ataxia type 3 and the purchase by Astellas (San Francisco) of Iveric Bio of New Jersey for $5.9 billion for programs on muscle disease and Pompe's disease.

The development of vaccines represents a special form of gene therapy and results from decades of basic and preclinical research, usually performed with both public funds and then by biotech and big Pharma funds. The development of the COVID-19 mRNA vaccines during the COVID pandemic of 2020–2023 is a scientifically and historically unique example of vaccine development from a base of publicly funded basic research and then by an unprecedented massive funding program by governmental and industrial sources. One major technical reason for the success of that program was in its use of technology and tools developed in the context of gene therapy, principally the application of the lipid nanoparticle gene transfer technology developed decades earlier by Philip Felgner at Vical in La Jolla, California. The combined mRNA basic research technology of Katalin Kariko and Drew Weissman at the University of Pennsylvania and the gene transfer tools developed by Felgner were the principal technologies that allowed the pharma and biotechnology firms Pfizer-BioNTech and Moderna to produce the conceptually new mRNA vaccines in a time period unheard of in the history of vaccine development cited by the award of Princess of Asturias Prize in 2022. Of course, the success of a vaccine must be proven in clinical testing, an achievement made possible for the COVID vaccines by the commitment of more than $30 billion, largely from the U.S. government "Warp Speed" COVID vaccine program.

The term "warp speed" might just as easily be applied to the ongoing explosion of biotechnology firms in the general area of genetic therapies. With the commercial impetus largely of the many new biotechnology firms appearing by the month, the field of gene-based therapy, including "traditional" virus vector–based techniques and now especially the rapidly maturing fields of genome editing by classical CRISPR-Cas9, base editing and prime editing are reaching technical maturity and clinical reality in times unimaginable just a few short years ago.

## Reference

1. Mullis K, Faloona F, Scharf S, Saiki R, Horn G, Erlich H. Specific enzymatic amplification of DNA in vitro: the polymerase chain reaction. In *Cold Spring Harbor symposia on quantitative biology*. Cold Spring Harbor Laboratory Press; 1986. PMID: 1422010.

# 22
# Current dilemma and future directions

It's not a great leap of imagination to see that the current and imminent advances in genetics will create immensely powerful tools for the prevention and treatment of human illness. We are already getting foretastes of how many of today's untreatable and even lethal diseases and physical, neurological and developmental defects will become distant memories and how yesterday's revolutionary discoveries of human anatomy, anesthesia, the germ theory, the development of antibiotics, vaccinology, modern pharmacology will pale in comparison to the effects of modern discoveries: science's ability to rewrite parts of the human genome and redirect some aspects of human evolution. This new era of genetic manipulation will redefine not only some of the core concepts of human biology but other elements of the entire biosphere, including nonhuman life, agriculture and biological evolutionary forces.

But it will not be a surprise if the future path of genetics is likely to be beset by scientific and ethical problems and that the application and misuse of manipulative genetics will generate many public policy dilemmas. The question of how those dilemmas will take shape and be resolved is unclear, but the existence of the uncertainties underscores the problem stated so eloquently by sages such as Niels Bohr and Yogi Berra and others—"making predictions is difficult, especially about the future."

Several areas are obvious troubling candidates for ethical and public policy concern; e.g., the current problem of increasingly prohibitive costs of gene-based therapies, the future problems surrounding the potential for human genetic enhancement, germ line manipulation and the potential for shaping human genetic future and evolution, the worrisome history of eugenics and the specter of its possible resurgence.

***Pricing.*** Accessibility and affordability remain troublesome problems for all advances in biomedicine, including gene-based therapies in all forms, whether they be traditional gene-transfer approaches or CRISPR-based genome editing applications. Gene therapy is one of the poster children of that problem, with announced prices for some recently approved gene therapies in the millions of dollars, ensuring that many patients will be unable to have needed therapies and that insurance companies will be unable or unwilling to cover or reimburse patients for such costs. A highly unsettling aspect of this commercial gene therapy frenzy is the resulting high cost of therapies that eventually reach the market and the high likelihood that many desperate patients will be priced out of their needed therapies. The rationales used to establish treatment costs seem at times to verge on a competition between biotech and pharmaceutical companies. The recently announced price by bluebird bio of $3 million for its newly approved gene therapy (Syskona) for cerebral adrenoleukodystrophy was greeted with almost breathless excitement that the price breaks bluebird's previous price record for treatment with Zynteglo for beta-thalassemia. The epochal development of gene-based therapies for intractable diseases is likely to be made increasingly complicated by costs and prices that put therapies out of reach of patients and that threaten the viability of the medical insurance structures. That problem cries out for combined industry-political-societal solutions.

***Eugenics.*** Eugenics has had a troubling history, from its earliest formulation by Francis Galton in the mid-to-late 19th century as a relatively innocuous means of encouraging socially beneficial matings to its more ignorant extension to exclusionary immigration policies and involuntary sterilization to its ultimate evil transformation in the Nazi genocidal programs in mid-20th century. The advent of CRISPR and other genome editing technologies has extended the original eugenic concept of Galton into the concept that human beings can and should be genetically modified toward the goal not merely to prevent and treat disease but also to enhance desirable human traits such as intelligence and socially "desirable" personality traits.

These concepts are not new, but what is qualitatively different now is the scientific basis for bringing some of these concepts close to reality. The scientific basis for early 20th-century eugenic thinking by the U.S. Supreme Court in the *Buck v. Bell* decision and in the Nazi genocidal programs was between nonexistent and poor, while the scientific basis for today's eugenics thinking is more solid, making it more likely that eugenic concepts will gain in credibility and popularity. Although previous versions of these issues were often flawed science, the current renewed concerns about these issues are warranted because the much greater strength of modern genetics makes these problems more likely to appear and to open the door to misadventures, mistakes and scientific and fatal hubris well known to the ancient Greeks. Daedalus crafted wings to enable his son Icarus to fly, but the wings were not strong enough to keep them from melting when Icarus flew too close to the sun. He plunged to his death, the victim not merely of failed technology but more so of human hubris. The lesson from Daedalus is that his hubris doomed Icarus to failure and to his death. Mary Shelley's Doctor Frankenstein fell victim to a similar fate.

*Therapy and enhancement.* In modern times, an industry of futurists has come to think about and even to urge the application of any scientific tools, including genetics, to enhance human traits and build an enhanced humanity. A major proponent of this approach has been Julian Savulescu of the University of Oxford who proposed that, "As a species, we have a moral obligation to enhance ourselves," including the design of genetically "improved" newborns and subsequent generations—more intelligent, longer-lived, more robust and forgiving personalities. Savulescu and other proponents of full-scale genetic human enhancement propose to save humanity from the vagaries of the capricious genetic lottery that has shaped us all and that has made all human beings appropriate targets for "improvement" and for redesign of humanity toward a better end.

A noble goal, but future applications of modern genetic wizardry and the search for "improved" and "enhanced" human beings not only will produce wonderful biomedical advances but are also likely to lead to inadvertent or even deliberate misadventure. One important dilemma that usually goes unresolved is the question of who and what kinds of social structures are needed to define what constitutes "improvement" and how the benefits of genetic enhancement are to be distributed and allocated. For that process to be ethically acceptable, one should require ideally that decisions and resource allocation be carried out behind a "veil of ignorance," as the American philosopher and ethicist John Rawls termed structures in which those who make ethical decisions or who determine allocation of benefits decide must not know if they are or are not beneficiaries of their decisions.

One area of concern is the temptation to apply genetic modification not only to specific individual human beings for specific disease traits but to use the tools of genetic modification to create "improved" and "enhanced" next generations, as through embryo and germ line genetic modification.

*Embryo and germ line modification.* As long as genetic modification of humans is limited to somatic cells and to individual subjects, there seem to be very few new ethical concerns that have not been faced with all other human interventions. But the potential to move genetic manipulation from somatic tissue and from treatment of individual patients to the germ line and to the genetic manipulation of future generations represents a completely new and troublesome capability based on firm scientific concepts, one for which human societies are currently technically, ethically or morally unprepared. Unfortunately, some social philosophers and academicians have supported the use of all means, including even embryonic and germ line genetic modification. But the potential for hubristic and unwise genetic manipulation is not merely theoretical—it has become a reality. It should have come as no surprise, and yet it was an unsettling shock that, in November 2018, the Chinese scientist He Jianjui announced at the Second International Human Genome Editing Summit in Hong Kong in the presence of many of the world's genome editing pioneers and thought leaders that he had carried out a CRISPR-Cas9 editing procedure on cultured human embryos in vitro with the intention of knocking out the receptor for HIV in those embryos and presumably making resulting live infants resistant to HIV infection. Of the genetically modified embryos, two implanted embryos advanced successfully through pregnancy to produce two live babies. Because his announcement flew in the face of previously established ethical, scientific and public policy guidelines for genome editing in general and for germ line genetic modification specifically, his announcement was met with a variety of generally harsh and unforgiving ethical, scientific and public policy critiques. He had apparently not carried out his studies according to required institutional and governmental protocols and had acted in defiance of Chinese legal constraints against embryo and germ line genetic modification. He suffered the loss of his faculty position and was imprisoned for three years. He has recently resumed some scientific work after admitting recently that he performed his embryo modification work "too early."

The overwhelmingly negative reaction to He's experiment from most of the scientific community has been underscored by formal scientific and policy statements from high-level national bodies such as the American Association for the Advancement of Science (AAAS) (1), United States National Academy of Sciences, the United States Institute of Medicine and the U.K. Royal Society (2, 3). In their prescient 2000 book *Human Inheritable Genetic Modifications (Assessing Scientific, Ethical, Religious, and Policy Issues)*, Frankel and Chapman recommended that, until the state of the underlying genetic science is much more advanced, a moratorium should be placed on germ line modification. A potential scientifically justifiable and ethically acceptable road to human genetic enhancement through embryo and germ line manipulation has not yet been identified, and the obstacles toward that end have recently been reviewed. Jennifer Doudna of the influential Innovative Genomics Institute (IGI) at the University of California Berkeley Institute has underscored that reservation by reaffirming that germ line genetic modification cannot be justified by today's science.

A definitive set of recommendations of the joint combined national academies (2, 3), published in 2020 in the aftermath of the 2018 He debacle and reproduced below, present a detailed and highly restrictive set of recommendations that underscore the depth of their concern about the potential threat to humanity of inappropriate human genetic editing. The broad recommendations and restrictions deserve to be considered to be formal guidelines for future attempts at heritable human genetic modification and are summarized in full in the attached Appendix.

### References

1. Frankel M, Chapman A. *Human Inheritable Genetic Modifications: Assessing Scientific, Ethical, Religious, and Policy Issues.* Washington, DC: AAAS Press; 2000.
2. Baltimore D, Berg P, Botchan M, Carroll D, Charo RA, Church G, Corn JE, Daley GQ, Doudna JA, Fenner M, Greely HT, Jinek M, Martin GS, Penhoet E, Puck J, Sternberg SH, Weissman JS, Yamamoto KR. Biotechnology. A prudent path forward for genomic engineering and germline gene modification. *Science.* 2015 Apr 3;348(6230):36–38. doi10.1126/science.aab1028. Epub 2015 Mar 19. PMID: 25791083.
3. Heritable Human Genome Editing, National Academy of Medicine, National Academy of Sciences, and the Royal Society. 2020. Heritable Human Genome Editing. Washington, DC: The National Academies Press. https://doi.org/10.17226/25665

## Appendix

## Heritable human genome editing. United States National Academy of Sciences, United States Institute of Medicine and U.K. Royal Society

**Recommendation 1:** No attempt to establish a pregnancy with a human embryo that has undergone genome editing should proceed unless and until it has been clearly established that it is possible to efficiently and reliably make precise genomic changes without undesired changes in human embryos. These criteria have not yet been met, and further research and review would be necessary to meet them.

**Recommendation 2:** Extensive societal dialogue should be undertaken before a country makes a decision on whether to permit clinical use of heritable human genome editing

(HHGE). The clinical use of HHGE raises not only scientific and medical considerations but also societal and ethical issues that were beyond the Commission's charge.

**Recommendation 3:** It is not possible to define a responsible translational pathway applicable across all possible uses of heritable human genome editing (HHGE) because the uses, circumstances, and considerations differ widely, as do the advances in fundamental knowledge that would be needed before different types of uses could be considered feasible.

Clinical use of HHGE should proceed incrementally. At all times, there should be clear thresholds on permitted uses, based on whether a responsible translational pathway can be and has been clearly defined for evaluating the safety and efficacy of the use, and whether a country has decided to permit the use.

**Recommendation 4:** Initial uses of heritable human genome editing (HHGE), should a country decide to permit them, should be limited to circumstances that meet all of the following criteria:

1. the use of HHGE is limited to serious monogenic diseases; the Commission defines a serious monogenic disease as one that causes severe morbidity or premature death;
2. the use of HHGE is limited to changing a pathogenic genetic variant known to be responsible for the serious monogenic disease to a sequence that is common in the relevant population and that is known not to be disease-causing;
3. no embryos without the disease-causing genotype will be subjected to the process of genome editing and transfer, to ensure that no individuals resulting from edited embryos were exposed to risks of HHGE without any potential benefit; and
4. the use of HHGE is limited to situations in which prospective parents: (i) have no option for having a genetically related child that does not have the serious monogenic disease, because none of their embryos would be genetically unaffected in the absence of genome editing, or (ii) have extremely poor options, because the expected proportion of unaffected embryos would be unusually low, which the Commission defines as 25% or less, and have attempted at least one cycle of preimplantation genetic testing without success.

**Recommendation 5:** Before any attempt to establish a pregnancy with an embryo that has undergone genome editing, preclinical evidence must demonstrate that heritable human genome editing (HHGE) can be performed with sufficiently high efficiency and precision to be clinically useful. For any initial uses of HHGE, preclinical evidence of safety and efficacy should be based on the study of a significant cohort of edited human embryos and should demonstrate that the process has the ability to generate and select, with high accuracy, suitable numbers of embryos that:

- have the intended edit(s) and no other modification at the target(s);
- lack additional variants introduced by the editing process at off-target sites—that is, the total number of new genomic variants should not differ significantly from that found in comparable unedited embryos;
- lack evidence of mosaicism introduced by the editing process;
- are of suitable clinical grade to establish a pregnancy; and
- have aneuploidy rates no higher than expected based on standard assisted reproductive technology procedures.

**Recommendation 6:** Any proposal for initial clinical use of heritable human genome editing should meet the criteria for preclinical evidence set forth in Recommendation 5. A proposal for clinical use should also include plans to evaluate human embryos prior to transfer using:

- developmental milestones until the blastocyst stage comparable with standard in vitro fertilization practices; and
- a biopsy at the blastocyst stage that demonstrates
  o the existence of the intended edit in all biopsied cells and no evidence of unintended edits at the target locus; and
  o no evidence of additional variants introduced by the editing process at off-target sites.

If, after rigorous evaluation, a regulatory approval for embryo transfer is granted, monitoring during a resulting pregnancy and long-term follow-up of resulting children and adults is vital.

**Recommendation 7:** Research should continue into the development of methods to produce functional human gametes from cultured stem cells. The ability to generate large numbers of such stem cell–derived gametes would provide a further option for prospective parents to avoid the inheritance of disease through the efficient production, testing, and selection of embryos without the disease-causing genotype. However, the use of such in vitro–derived gametes in reproductive medicine raises distinct medical, ethical, and societal issues that must be carefully evaluated, and such gametes without genome editing would need to be approved for use in assisted reproductive technology before they could be considered for clinical use of heritable human genome editing.

**Recommendation 8:** Any country in which the clinical use of heritable human genome editing (HHGE) is being considered should have mechanisms and competent regulatory bodies to ensure that all of the following conditions are met:

- individuals conducting HHGE-related activities, and their oversight bodies, adhere to established principles of human rights, bioethics, and global governance;
- the clinical pathway for HHGE incorporates best practices from related technologies such as mitochondrial replacement techniques, preimplantation genetic testing, and somatic genome editing;
- decision-making is informed by findings from independent international assessments of progress in scientific research and the safety and efficacy of HHGE, which indicate that the technologies are advanced to a point that they could be considered for clinical use;
- prospective review of the science and ethics of any application to use HHGE is diligently performed by an appropriate body or process, with decisions made on a case-by-case basis;
- notice of proposed applications of HHGE being considered is provided by an appropriate body;
- details of approved applications (including genetic condition, laboratory procedures, laboratory or clinic where this will be done, and national bodies providing oversight) are made publicly accessible, while protecting family identities;
- detailed procedures and outcomes are published in peer-reviewed journals to provide dissemination of knowledge that will advance the field;

- the norms of responsible scientific conduct by individual investigators and laboratories are enforced;
- researchers and clinicians show leadership by organizing and participating in open international discussions on the coordination and sharing of results of relevant scientific, clinical, ethical, and societal developments impacting the assessment of HHGE's safety, efficacy, long-term monitoring, and societal acceptability;
- practice guidelines, standards, and policies for clinical uses of HHGE are created and adopted prior to offering clinical use of HHGE; and
- reports of deviation from established guidelines are received and reviewed, and sanctions are imposed where appropriate.

**Recommendation 9:** An International Scientific Advisory Panel (ISAP) should be established with clear roles and responsibilities before any clinical use of heritable human genome editing (HHGE). The ISAP should have a diverse, multidisciplinary membership and should include independent experts who can assess scientific evidence of safety and efficacy of both genome editing and associated assisted reproductive technologies. The ISAP should:

- provide regular updates on advances in, and the evaluation of, the technologies that HHGE would depend on and recommend further research developments that would be required to reach technical or translational milestones;
- assess whether preclinical requirements have been met for any circumstances in which HHGE may be considered for clinical use;
- review data on clinical outcomes from any regulated uses of HHGE and advise on the scientific and clinical risks and potential benefits of possible further applications; and
- provide input and advice on any responsible translational pathway to the international body described in Recommendation 10, as well as at the request of national regulators.

**Recommendation 10:** In order to proceed with applications of heritable human genome editing (HHGE) that go beyond the translational pathway defined for initial classes of use of HHGE, an international body with appropriate standing and diverse expertise and experience should evaluate and make recommendations concerning any proposed new class of use.

This international body should:

- clearly define each proposed new class of use and its limitations;
- enable and convene ongoing transparent discussions on the societal issues surrounding the new class of use;
- make recommendations concerning whether it could be appropriate to cross the threshold of permitting the new class of use; and
- provide a responsible translational pathway for the new class of use.

**Recommendation 11:** An international mechanism should be established by which concerns about research or conduct of heritable human genome editing that deviates from established guidelines or recommended standards can be received, transmitted to relevant national authorities, and publicly disclosed.

# 23

# Summary: genetic therapies—a new field of medicine

The birth and early development of gene-based therapies have represented modern equivalents of some of the most revolutionary discoveries in the history of medicine. Perhaps the most important and earliest of the modern changes was the discovery that under some conditions, exposure to a disease-causing agent can produce a beneficial immune response that will not only prevent development of clinical disease but that will also protect exposed healthy people from future disease by that agent. In 1796, Edward Jenner intuited that some people, notably milkmaids, were protected from developing smallpox because of their prior exposure to pustules on cows infected with cowpox. That discovery was the birth of vaccination. The invention of the microscope by van Leeuwenhoek and Robert Hooke in the 17th century (1632–1723) led to the formulation by Schleiden, Schwann and Virchow in the 19th century, who established the cell as the underlying structural unit of all living matter. Louis Pasteur and Robert Koch established the principles of the germ theory of disease, and this birth of microbiology together with the invention in mid-19th century of anesthesia by William Morton and antisepsis by Joseph Lister and Ignaz Semmelweiss later in the 19th century produced the art and technical marvels of surgery.

The addition of modern genetics and gene-based therapies to this list of marvels was made possible of course by the discovery of the principles and laws of genetics by Charles Darwin, Gregor Mendel, Archibald Garrod and the many giants who gave birth to molecular and human genetics—Thomas Morgan, Barbara McClintock, Oswald Avery, James Watson, Francis Crick, Sydney Brenner, Rosalind Franklin, Jacques Monod, Francois Jacob, Werner Arber, Daniel Nathans, Hamilton Smith, Paul Berg, David Baltimore, Howard Temin, Fred Sanger and, most recently, Emmanuelle Charpentier and Jennifer Doudna.

The discoveries and principles laid out by these scientists have made possible the remarkable new concept of gene-based therapy for human disease, using either the now "traditional" gene therapy tools of vector-mediated gene transfer and increasingly the more recently developed tools of gene editing. This new approach to therapy represents a qualitative leap from all previous therapies because it is designed to correct rather than merely to circumvent the effects of the underlying genetic aberration. There is no doubt that, even at the current early stage of the development of gene therapies, gene therapy has become a legitimate new field of medicine and has begun to provide effective treatment for a growing number of diseases, particularly single-gene Mendelian diseases and, in the form of CAR-T therapy, for several hematological malignancies.

But the advent of gene editing, for both DNA and RNA reprogramming, promises to change everything. The field of gene-based therapy is on the cusp of being able to bring about permanent definitive correction of disease-related genetic defects by a reprogramming edit of aberrant genetic information. In the remarkably short period of little more than one decade, zinc-finger and TALEN editing have both shown proof of concept and clinical promise for the prevention of infectious disease such as HIV and for the successful treatment of a case of relapsed leukemia. Even more impressive is the fact that in less than ten years since its discovery, CRISPR-based editing has shown proof of concept for treatment of sickle cell anemia and beta-thalassemia.

That rapid development is both encouraging and also a warning that the technology of human genetic modification is accelerating beyond the state of scientific and ethical preparedness. In less than 4 years after the initial reports of CRISPR-Cas9 genome editing, a disturbing application was undertaken by an investigator in China to use CRISPR-Cas9 editing tools to edit HIV receptors in human embryos. The "experiment" was a scientific and ethical disaster and underscored the fact the genetic editing had become technically so accessible to qualified and unqualified investigators that disreputable and unethical applications were inevitable. Formal guidelines and declarations of principles have been and will continue to be developed, but the ease of genetic manipulations, even with today's first-stage genetic editing tools ensures that poorly designed applications, misadventures, mistakes and harm will ensue.

Equally concerning is the fact that the availability of such effective genetic tools will underscore the dilemma of what genetic traits should be considered suitable targets for genetic modification. What is the distinction between legitimately targeted "disease" traits and normal human traits whose genetics is a tempting target for modification? Might the mere existence of some kinds of favored and genetically modified humans per se create a class of un-favored human beings not eligible for the medical wonders of the genetic revolution? When, how and by whom should the decisions be made for identifying the appropriate participants in these genetic wonders? How can our society best be prepared for the benefits of this technological revolution, and how can it be protected from the potential and the inevitable missteps and misadventures? At the dawn of genetic therapies during the early and late 20th century, the eventual development of the current descriptive and manipulative applications of genetic science was far beyond our imagination. But we are in the midst of the reality of that revolution and are already beginning to catch a glimpse of the boundless good and some unsettling dangers of human genetic modification. Our current new era of gene-based therapies and human genetic modification call for major societal educational programs for preparing the public to deal with such complex questions.

# Index

*For the benefit of digital users, indexed terms that span two pages (e.g., 52–53) may, on occasion, appear on only one of those pages.*

Page references followed by *f* denote figures.

AAAS (American Association for the Advancement of Science), 184–85
AAV (adeno-associated virus) vectors, 112–15, 119, 149–50, 179
Abbas, Haly (Ali Iban Abbas), 9
ABCD1 gene, 156
academia, 141, 175, 179–80
Acland, Gregory, 147–48
acute lymphoblastic leukemia, 145
ADA (adenosine deaminase) deficiency, 120–22, 178
adeno-associated virus (AAV) vectors, 112–15, 119, 149–50, 179
adenosine deaminase (ADA) deficiency, 120–22, 146–47, 178
adenosine phosphoribosyltransferase (aprt) gene transfer, 86–87
adenovirus vectors, 107–8, 142
Advexin, 142
Aesculapius (Asklepios), 3–5, 4*f*
Aiuti, Allessandro, 146*f*, 146–47
Al-Baghdadi, 9
albinism, 31–34
Alcmaeon, 3–4
alkaptonuria, 31–34, 33*f*
Allogene, Inc., 159
Al-Razi (Razes), 9
American Association for the Advancement of Science (AAAS), 184–85
American Society of Gene Therapy, 139
Amsterdam Molecular Therapeutics (AMT), 178–79
amyloidosis, transthyretin, 165–66
amyotrophic lateral sclerosis (ALS), 172–73, 179–80
anatomy, 9–10
ancient Greeks, 3–4
Anderson, William French, 95, 96*f*, 120, 121, 135–36, 178
anesthesia, 189

angioedema, 165–66
animalcules, 10, 13*f*
anthrax, 18
antigen escape, 151–52
antisense synthetic oligonucleotides (ASOs), 171–73
Aposhian, Vasken, 64–65
Arber, Werner, 73–77, 75*f*, 189
Aristotle, 17
arthritis, 31–34
aseptic surgery, 19
Asilomar conferences, 91–95
ASOs (antisense synthetic oligonucleotides), 171–73
Astellas, 179–80
astronomy, 9
Atchison, Robert, 112–13
ATTR amyloidosis (life-threatening transthyretin amyloidosis), 165–66
Avery, Oswald, 41–42, 44*f*, 189

bacterial viruses (phages or bacteriophages), 61, 81*f*
 DNA phage T2, 43–46
 lambda phage, 76–77
Al-Baghdadi, 9
Baltimore, David, 77–79, 79*f*, 108–10, 189
Banbury Center, 110, 111*f*
Banting, Frederick, 35*f*, 35–36
base editing, 166–67, 173–74
Bateson, William, 31, 32*f*
Batshaw, Mark, 135–37
B-cell leukemia, 151–52
B-cell lymphoma, 151–52, 159
BCL11A gene, 158–59
Beadle, George, 42–43, 45*f*
Beecher, Henry, 127–28
Belmont report, 129
Bennett, Jean, 147–48, 148*f*, 149*f*
Berg, Paul, 76*f*, 76–77, 79–81, 91–92, 92*f*, 189

Berra, Yogi, 181
Best, Charles, 35f, 35–36
beta-thalassemia, 87–89, 158–59
   CRISPR clinical trials, 164–65
   treatment of, 164–65, 181–82, 190
betibeglogene autotemcel, 164–65
big pharma, 179–80
Biogen, 177, 179–80
BioMarin, Inc., 179
biotechnology (biotech), 81–84, 164, 175–80
Birndorf, Howard, 177
blindness, congenital, 147–48
blood circulation, 10, 13f
bluebird bio, 156, 164–65, 181–82
Bohr, Niels, 181
bone sarcoma, metastatic, 163–64
Bordignon, Claudio, 146–47
Boveri, Theodor, 37
Boyer, Herbert, 77f, 77, 81–84, 176
Boyle, Robert, 10–15
Boyle's Law, 10–15
Brenner, Sydney, 67, 71f, 155, 189
Briard dogs, 147–48
Broad Institute, 161–62
Brown, Michael, 54f
Buck, Carrie, 23–24
*Buck v. Bell*, 23–24, 128, 182–83

calcium phosphate gene transfer, 87–89, 99
California Institute of Technology (Caltech), 38–39
Cambridge University, 51f, 56–57, 67, 79–81
cancer
   gene therapy for, 142–43, 151–52
   head and neck, 142–43
   hematological, 159
   immunotherapy for, 151–52, 175–76
   non-small cell lung cancer, 163
Capecchi, Mario, 157
capsid G protein, 110–12
Carnegie Institution, 43–46
Carter, Barrie, 113, 115f
Cas endonucleases (CRISPR-associated proteins), 160
   Cas9, 160–63, 165–66, 173–74
   Cas12, 173–74
   Cas13, 173–74
cationic lipid reagents, 99–101, 177
Celera Genomics, 132–33
cell theory, 9–20, 14f, 189
central nervous system (CNS) gene therapy, 179–80
cerebral leukodystrophy, 156
cervical intraepithelial neoplasia, 159
Cetus Corp., 175–76

CGD (chronic granulomatous disease), 147
Chandrasegaran, Srinivasan, 158
Chargaff, Erwin, 47–48
Chargaff rules, 47–50
Charpentier, Emmanuelle, 161–62, 162f, 189
Chase, Martha, 45–47, 48f
chemical nonviral vectors, 99–104
chimeric antigen receptor (CAR) T-cells, 150–52, 159, 189–90
China
   clinical trials, 142–43, 163–66
   Food and Drug Administration (CFDA), 142
cholera, 18
cholesterol metabolism, 53
chromosomes, 37, 38–39, 41
   description of, 37–40
   Sutton-Boveri theory, 37–40
chronic granulomatous disease (CGD), 147, 167
City of Hope Hospital (Duarte, California), 81–84, 176–77
Claudius Galenus. *See* Galen
Cline, Martin, 87–89, 88f, 129–30, 139
clinical genetics, 59–60
clinical trials
   CRISPR, 163–66
   design of, 127–30
   ethical principles, 129, 138–39
   gene therapy trials, 87–89, 95, 107–8, 108f, 119–25, 129–30, 138–39, 143–47, 144f, 149f, 150f, 178
   gene transfer trials, 156
   phase I, 120, 159, 163–64
   phase II, 129–30
   phase III, 129–30, 172–73
   randomized controlled trials (RCTs), 127, 129–30
cloning, 81–84
clotting factors, 81–84
clustered regularly interspaced short palindromic repeats. *See* CRISPR
Cohen, Stanley, 77f, 77
Cold Spring Harbor Laboratory, 24, 39–40, 43–47, 71f, 112f, 131–32
   Banbury Center, 110, 111f
   Eugenics Record Office, 21–23
Collins, Francis, 131–32, 132f
Collip, James, 35–36
Columbia University, 38–39
complementary DNA (cDNA), 81–84, 88–89, 120
Cooperative Research and Development agreement (CRADA), 120
Copernicus, Nicolaus, 9
Corey, Robert, 48–50

Cornell University, 147–48
Correns, Karl Franz Joseph, 28f, 28
Cotton, Matthew (Matt), 101, 102f
COVID-19 mRNA vaccines, 179–80
COVID pandemic, 99–101
coxsackie viruses, 115
Crick, Francis, 49–51, 51f, 67–68, 71f, 189
CRISPR (clustered regularly interspaced short palindromic repeats)
 -based editing, 163–66, 190
 -based therapy, 165–66
 -Cas9 editing, 160–63, 166, 173–74
 clinical trials, 163–66
 -modulated genome editing, 171
 RNA-guided nucleases, 157–58
 terminology, 160
CRISPR-associated proteins (Cas endonucleases), 160
 Cas9, 160–63, 165–66, 173–74
 Cas12, 173–74
 Cas13, 173–74
CRISPR Therapeutics, 164–65
crossing-over, 38–39
CSL Behring, 179
C-to-U RNA editor (CURE) editing, 173–74
CTX001, 165
Culver, Kenneth, 122f
CURE (C-to-U RNA editor) editing, 173–74
Cure Rare Disease (CRD), 165–66
current dilemma, 181–88
cyclin-dependent kinase 2A gene *(CDKN2A)*, 145
cystic fibrosis, 129, 159
cystinuria, 31–34

Daedalus, 182–83
Dan David Prize, 151–52
Darwin, Charles, 21, 24–28, 189
Davenport, Charles, 21–23
DEAE (diethylaminoethyl)-dextran, 85, 99
deletions, 160
DeLisi, Charles, 131–32
dementia, frontotemporal (FTD), 172–73, 179–80
de Vries, Hugo Marie, 24–27, 37–38
diabetes mellitus, 34
 insulin therapy for, 35–36, 176–77
 type I, 34
 type II, 34
diabetic retinopathy, 173
diethylaminoethyl (DEAE)-dextran, 85, 99
N-[1-(2,3-dioleyloxy)propyl]- N,N,N- trimethylammonium chloride (DOTMA) (lipofectin), 99
disease
 early Western concepts of, 3–8

 genetic, 59f, 59–60
 genetic basis of, 41
 germ theory of, 17, 189
 molecular, 53–60
 mutation-induced, 37
disinfection, 19
DNA
 base components, 47–48
 complementary DNA (cDNA), 81–84
 discovery of, 41–42, 46–48
 images of, 49f, 49–50
 recombinant, 67–84, 91–97, 176–77
 research oversight and regulation, 91–97
 sequencing, 79–84, 81f, 83f
 structure of, 47–51, 55f
 SV-40-based recombinant DNA gene transfer vector, 76–77
DNA phage T2, 43–46
DNA polymerase I, 67
DOTMA (N-[1-(2,3-dioleyloxy)propyl]- N,N,N- trimethylammonium chloride) (lipofectin), 99
double-strand breaks (DSB), 158
Doudna, Jennifer, 161f, 161–62, 184–85, 189
*Drosophila melanogaster*, 37–39
Duchenne muscular atrophy, 150f
Dulbecco, Renato, 63, 68–69, 73f, 76–77, 105–6, 131–32

Editas Medicine, 164
Egyptian medicine, 3–4
electroporation, 85–86
Eli Lilly Inc., 176–77
elivaldogene autotemcel (Skysona), 156
embryo and germ line modification, 183–85
England, 131–32
enhancement, 183
enteroviruses, recombinant, 115
enzymes, restriction, 70–77
epidermolysis bullosum, 159
*Escherichia coli*, 46–47, 77, 91–92, 176–77
Eshhar, Zelig, 151
ethical concerns
 conflicts of interest, 138
 current dilemmas, 182–85, 190–91
 informed consent, 89, 129
 President's Commission for the Study of Ethical Problems in Medicine and Biomedical and Behavioral Research, 95, 119–20
 requirements for human experimentation, 129, 138–39
eugenics, 21–24, 182–83
Europe, 129–30

European Medicines Agency (EMA)
  clinical trials, 129–30, 156, 163–66
  gene therapies approved by, 142, 149–50, 164–65, 178–79
evidence-based medicine, 5–6
eye disease, 147–48, 172, 173
Eylea, 173

factor IX-deficiency hemophilia, 156
*Federal Register*, 93–94, 95
Felgner, Philip (Phil), 99, 100f, 101–3, 177, 179–80
Fenzl, Eduard, 27–28
fetal hemoglobin (HbF), 158–59, 164
fever, puerperal, 19–20
Fischer, Alain, 105–6, 143–45, 144f
fly room (Columbia University), 38–39
foamy virus (FV) retroviruses, 115
Fok I restriction endonuclease, 158
Food and Drug Administration (CFDA or CSFDA) (China), 142
Food and Drug Administration (FDA) (U.S.)
  clinical trials, 129–30, 138–39, 156, 167, 172–73
  CRISPR-based therapies approved by, 165–66
  gene therapies approved by, 142, 149–50, 179
  RNA-based therapies approved by, 172
  synthetic insulin approved by, 176–77
  synthetic recombinant human growth hormone approved by, 176–77
France, 131–32
Frankenstein, 182–83
Franklin, Rosalind, 49f, 49–50, 189
Frederickson, Donald, 93f, 93–94
French Muscular Dystrophy Association, 177–78
Friedmann, Theodore, 69–70, 74f, 75f, 81f, 105–6, 106f, 110
frontotemporal dementia (FTD), 172–73, 179–80
future directions, 181–88

Galen, 3–4, 6–7, 7f, 9
Galileo Galilei, 9
Galton, Francis, 21–23, 23f, 182
gammaretrovirus vectors, 119, 120, 146–47
Garrod, Archibald, 29–30, 31–36, 32f, 33f, 141–42, 189
Gaucher's Disease, 159
Gelsinger, Jesse, 107–8, 108f, 135–38, 136f, 139
Gendicine, 142
gene (term), 37

gene-based therapy. *See* gene therapy
gene editing, 155–69
  base editing, 166–67, 173–74
  CRISPR-based, 163–66, 190
  CRISPR-Cas9, 160–63, 166, 173–74
  C-to-U RNA editor (CURE) editing, 173–74
  current dilemmas, 183
  development of, 189–90
  ethical concerns, 190–91
  future directions, 190–91
  guidelines for, 190
  prime editing, 166, 167, 173–74
  programmable RNA-based RNA editing, 173–74
  recommendations on, 185–88
  RNA editing for programmable adenosine replacement (REPAIR), 173–74
  RNA editing for specific C-to-U exchange (RESCUE), 173–74
  RNA editing tools and targets, 171–73
  techniques, 166
  zinc (Zn)-finger base editing, 166–67, 190
gene expression, 39–40
Genentech, Inc., 77f, 81–84, 173, 176–77
genes, 24–27, 37–40, 41
gene splicing, 73–76, 81–84
gene therapy, 31–34
  ASO oligonucleotide-based, 171–73
  for beta-thalassemia, 164–65, 181–82, 190
  breakthrough, 141–54
  clinical proof of principle, 105–6, 176
  clinical trials, 87–89, 95, 107–8, 108f, 119–25, 129–30, 143–47, 144f, 149f, 150f, 178
  current dilemmas, 181–82, 183
  development of, 105–6, 175–80, 189–90
  emergence of, 1–2
  first licensed product, 142, 178–79
  future directions, 181–82
  gene editing, 155–69
  history of, 61–65, 75f, 105–17, 119–25
  immunotherapy as, 150–52
  OTC trials, 107–8, 108f, 135–37
  *Points to Consider in the Design and Submission of Somatic Cell Human Gene Therapy Protocols*, 95
  pricing, 181–82
  product replacement approach, 34–36, 141–42
  RNA-based therapies, 171–74
  for SCID, 122–23, 129–30, 143–47, 144f, 178
  setbacks, 135–39
  summary, 189–91
  traditional applications, 151

traditional approaches, 155–57
traditional tools, 189–90
vector-mediated, 189–90
*Gene Therapy: A Handbook for Physicians* (Culver), 122*f*
Gene Therapy Center, University of Pennsylvania, 135–39
*Gene Therapy: Fact and Fiction* (Friedmann), 110, 111*f*
Gene Therapy Inc., 120
Genethon, 177–78
genetic diseases
　recognition of, 59*f*, 59–60
　treatment of, 141–42
genetic engineering, 81–84, 95
genetic modification, 183, 185–88
genetics
　biochemical, 31–36
　birthplace of, 24, 26*f*
　DNA as repository and transmitter of information, 41–42, 46–47
　history of, 21–30, 31–36, 105–17
　medical, 57, 58*f*
　molecular, 53–60
Genetic Therapy Inc. (GTI), 178
genetic transduction, 91
genetic transposition, 39–40, 40*f*
gene transfer
　cationic lipid reagents for, 99–101
　classical methods, 156
　federal oversight and regulation of, 85–90
　history of, 86–87
gene transfer vectors
　adeno-associated virus (AAV), 112–15, 119, 149–50, 179
　adenovirus, 107–8, 142
　chemical nonviral, 99–104
　lentivirus, 108–12
　retrovirus, 108–12, 151
　virus-based, 61–65, 70, 76–77, 105–6, 115
genocide, 182–83
genome editing, 156–58
　CRISPR-Cas9, 160–63, 166, 173–74
　CRISPR-modulated, 171
　recommendations for future attempts, 185–88
　techniques, 166
　zinc (Zn)-finger, 158–59
genotoxicity, 114–15, 146–47
genotype (term), 24–27, 37
Genovo, Inc., 136–37, 138
Germany
　Human Genome Project, 131–32

Nazi, 24, 128, 182–83
germ line modification, 183–85
germ theory, 17, 189
Gilbert, Walter, 76–77, 79–81, 80*f*, 131, 177
GlaxoSmithKline (GSK), 147, 179–80
Glybera, 178–79
Goldstein, Joseph, 54*f*
Gordon Conference on Nucleic Acids, 91–92
Graham, Frank, 86*f*, 86–87
Great Ormond Street Hospital (London), 143–45, 159
Greece, 3–4
Griffith, Frederick, 41, 42*f*
Griffith Experiment, 41, 42*f*, 43*f*
GTI (Genetic Therapy Inc.), 178

Haldane, J.B.S., 38–39
Hamer, Dean, 106–7
handwashing, 19–20
Harvard University, 73–76, 79–81, 122–23, 127–28, 166
Harvey, William, 6–7, 10, 13*f*
Hauswirth, William, 147–48
head and neck cancer, 142–43
He Jianjui, 183–85
Helsinki Declaration, 129
hematological cancers, 159
hematopoietic stem cells (HPSCs), 164–65
Hemgenix (CSL Behring), 156, 179
hemoglobin, 53–54
　fetal (HbF), 158–59, 164
　sickle cell (Hb-S), 54–57
hemophilia, factor IX-deficiency, 156
hemophilia A, 81–84, 179
hemophilia B, 81–84, 158–59, 179
hepatitis, 128, 129
hepatitis B, 177
herbal cures, 9
heritable human genome editing (HHGE). *See* genome editing
herpes simplex, 86–87
herpes viruses, 115
Hershey, Alfred, 43–47, 47*f*
Hippocrates, 3–6, 5*f*, 8
Hippocratic Corpus, 6
Hippocratic Oath, 6
HIV infection
　CRISPR-Cas9-based studies, 166
　therapy and prevention of, 158, 183–84
HIV virus, 108–9, 110–12
Holley, Robert, 52
Holmes, Oliver Wendel, 23–24
homogentisic acid, 31–34

homologous recombination (HR), 157–58
homology-directed repair (HDR), 160
Hooke, Robert, 10–15, 14f, 189
HPRT (hypoxanthine-guanine phosphoribosyltransferase)-deficiency Lesch–Nyhan disease, 105–6, 110
HPV (human papillomavirus), 159
Human Gene Therapy Subcommittee (HGTS), 95
human genetics
  biochemical, 31–36
  history of, 189
  *See also* genetics
Human Genome Consortium, 79–81
Human Genome Program (NIH), 131–32
Human Genome Project, 131–33, 177–78
human growth hormone, synthetic recombinant, 176–77
human papillomavirus (HPV), 159
Human Stem Cells Institute (Russia), 143
Humulin (insulin), 176–77
Huntington's disease, 179–80
Hybridtech Inc., 177
hydrodynamic delivery, 101–3
hypercholesterolemia, 53
hypoxanthine-guanine phosphoribosyltransferase (HPRT)-deficiency Lesch–Nyhan disease, 105–6, 110

Ibn Abbas, Ali (Haly Abbas), 9
Icarus, 182–83
iduronate 2-sulfatase (IDS) gene, 158–59
α-l-iduronidase (IDUA) gene, 158–59
IGI (Innovative Genomics Institute), 184–85
immunogenicity, 107–8
immunotherapy, 150–52, 175–76
improvement, 183
inborn errors of metabolism, 31–34, 33f, 36, 57
indels (insertions or deletions), 160
infectious disease, 18, 19–20
informed consent, 89, 129
Ingram, Vernon, 54–57, 57f
inheritance
  laws of, 24–30, 31–34, 37, 41
  *Mendelian Inheritance in Man* (MIM) (McKusick), 57–60, 58f, 59f
  of mutations, 37
  Online Mendelian Inheritance in Man (OMIM), 59f, 59–60
Innovative Genomics Institute (IGI), 184–85
inoculation, 15–17
insertions or deletions (indels), 160

Institute of Medicine (U.S.), 185–88
insulin
  discovery of, 34–36
  synthetic, 81–84, 176–77
insulin deficiency, 34
insulin therapy, 35–36, 176–77
Intellia Therapeutics, 165–66
interferon, 175–76
International Human Genome Editing Summit (2018), 183–84
International Scientific Advisory Panel (ISAP) (recommendation), 188
Introgen, 142
Isaiah, 63
ISAP (International Scientific Advisory Panel) (recommendation), 188
Ishino, Y., 160
Islamic medicine, 9
Itakura, Keiichi, 81–84, 176
Itano, Harvey, 53–54
Iveric Bio, 179–80

Jacob, Francois, 67, 70f, 189
Japan, 131–32
Japan Prize, 105–6
Jenner, Edward, 15–17, 16f, 189
Johansen, Wilhelm, 24–27, 37
Johns Hopkins University, 57, 73–76, 158
  Online Mendelian Inheritance in Man (OMIM), 59f, 59–60
  Welch Medical Library, 59f, 59–60
*Journal of Biological Chemistry*, 111f
June, Carl, 151–52, 153f

Kariko, Katalin, 99–101, 101f, 179–80
Khorana, Gobind, 52
Kleiner, Perkins, Caufield and Byers, 176
Klug, Aaron, 158
Koch, Robert, 15, 18f, 18, 189
Koch postulates, 18
Kornberg, Arthur, 67, 68f
Kurosawa, Yoshikazu, 151
Kyushu University, 160

Laboratory of Molecular Biology (LMB), 51f, 56–57, 67, 79–81, 158
Lamarck, Jean-Baptiste, 24–27
lambda phage, 76–77
large B-cell lymphoma (LBCL), 159
Laughlin, Harry, 21–23, 24
laws of inheritance, 37, 41
  discovery of, 24–30
  rediscovery of, 31–34

Leber's congenital amaurosis (LCA), 179
   AAV virus–mediated gene transfer trials, 147–48, 149f
   CRISPR clinical trials, 164
Leder, Philip, 106–7
Lederberg, Joshua, 91, 105
LentiGlobin (Zynteglo), 164–65
lentivirus vectors, 108–12, 164–65
Leonardo da Vinci, 10, 11f
Lesch-Nyhan disease, 105–6, 110
leukemia
   B-cell, 151–52
   T-cell, 145
leukodystrophy, cerebral, 156
life-threatening transthyretin amyloidosis (ATTR amyloidosis), 165–66
Li-Fraumeni Syndrome, 142
limey (term), 127
Lind, James, 127
linkage, 38–39
lipofectin (DOTMA), 99
lipofection technique, 99–101
Lister, Joseph, 15, 19f, 19, 189
Liu, David, 166, 167
LMB (Laboratory of Molecular Biology), 51f, 56–57, 67, 79–81
LMO2, 145
LocusBiosciences, 166
low-density lipoprotein (LDL), 53
Lu, You, 163
Lucentis, 173
lung cancer, non-small cell, 163
Luxturna (Spark Therapeutics Inc.), 179
lymphoma, B-cell, 151–52, 159

MacLeod, Colin, 41, 44f
Macleod, James, 35–36
Macugen, 173
macular degeneration, 173
maize, 39–40, 40f
mammalian papova viruses, 61
Marshall, Geoffrey, 129
Massachusetts Institute of Technology (MIT), 77–78, 91–92, 109–10, 161–62
Matthaei, Heinrich, 51, 52f
Maxam, Alan, 79–81
Max Planck Institute for Infection Biology (Berlin), 161–62
McCarty, Maclyn, 41–42, 45f
McClintock, Barbara, 39f, 39–40, 189
McKusick, Victor, 57–60, 58f
*The Mechanism of Mendelian Heredity* (Morgan), 38–39

medical genetics, 57, 58f
Medical Research Council (MRC), 56–57, 67, 129
Mendel, Gregor, 24–28, 25f, 41, 189
*Mendelian Inheritance in Man* (MIM) (McKusick), 59–60
   Online Mendelian Inheritance in Man (OMIM), 59f, 59–60
   print editions, 57–59, 58f
Mendell, Jerry, 149–50, 150f
Mendel's laws of inheritance
   discovery of, 24–30
   rediscovery of, 31–36
mercury, 9
Meselson, Matthew, 73–76
messenger RNA (mRNA), 51, 67–68, 171–72
   mRNA-based vaccines, 99–101, 179–80
metastatic bone sarcoma, 163–64
Michelangelo Buonarroti, 10, 12f
microbiology, 17, 19–20, 189
*Micrographia* (Hooke), 10–15
microorganisms, 10
microscopy, 10–15, 14f
Middle Ages, 9
MIT (Massachusetts Institute of Technology), 77–78, 91–92, 109–10, 161–62
Mizutani, Satoshi, 77–78
MLV (murine leukemia virus), 79, 108–9, 143–45
Moderna, 99–101, 179–80
Mojica, Francis, 160
Mok, Tony, 163
molecular biology
   central dogma, 67–68, 71f, 72f, 77–79
   history of, 67–84
molecular disease, 53–60, 55f, 56f
molecular genetics, 53–60, 189
MolMed, 147
Monod, Jacques, 67, 70f, 189
Morgan (unit), 38–39
Morgan, Thomas Hunt, 37–40, 38f, 189
Morton, William, 189
Motulsky, Arno, 122–24, 123f
mucopolysaccharidosis type I, 158–59
mucopolysaccharidosis type II, 158–59
Mullis, Karry, 175–76
murine leukemia virus (MLV), 79, 108–9, 143–45
muscle disease, 179–80
muscular dystrophy
   CRISPR clinical trials, 165–66
   Duchenne, 150f
   treatment of, 177–78

Muslim world, 9
mutations
  discovery of, 24–27
  inheritance of, 37
  mechanisms of, 42–43
  terminology, 24–27
Muzyczka, Nicholas (Nick), 113, 116f
myeloma, 163–64

Nägeli, Karl, 28
naked plasmid DNA, 101–3
Naldini, Luigi, 110–12, 114f, 146–47
Nathans, Daniel, 73–77, 75f, 189
National Academy of Sciences
  (US), 184–88
National Commission for the Protection
  of Human Subjects of Biomedical and
  Behavioral Research (US), 129
National Institutes of Health (NIH) (US), 51,
  67, 106–7, 109–10, 113
  1976 Director's meeting on recombinant
    DNA research, 92f
  gene therapy trials, 89, 119–24, 129–30,
    138–39, 178
  *Guidelines for Research Involving
    Recombinant DNA Molecules*, 93–94, 95
  Human Genome Program, 131–32
  patents, 121
  *Points to Consider in the Design and
    Submission of Somatic Cell Human Gene
    Therapy Protocols*, 95, 119
  Recombinant DNA Advisory Committee
    (RAC), 93–95, 119
  *Report and Recommendations of the Panel to
    Assess the NIH Investment in Research on
    Gene Therapy*, 122–24
Natural Science Society (Brno), 24
*Nature*, 49–50, 61–62, 79
Nazi Germany, 24, 128, 182–83
Nebuchadnezzar, 127
Necker Hospital (Paris, France), 143–45
Neumann, Eberhard, 85–86
*Neurospora crassa*, 42–43
*NIH Guidelines for Research Involving
  Recombinant DNA Molecules*, 93–94, 95
Nirenberg, Marshall, 51, 52f, 57f
Nobel Prize in Chemistry, 76–77, 79–81,
  82f, 161–62
Nobel Prize in Medicine or Physiology, 35–36,
  38–40, 46–47, 76–77, 79, 157, 175–76
non-homologous end joining (NHEJ), 157–
  58, 160
*NOTCH1* gene, 145
Novartis Gene Therapies, Inc., 179–80

nucleoside-modified mRNA-encoding viral
  antigens, 99–101
Nuremberg Code, 129
nusinersen (Spinraza), 172

Oak Right National Laboratory (US), 61–62
obstetrical infections, 19–20
Ochoa, Severo, 67, 69f
*Oenothera lamarckia*, 24–27
off-target effects, 162
Ohio State University, 149–50
oligonucleotides
  antisense synthetic (ASOs), 171–73
  small interfering RNA (siRNA), 173
Online Mendelian Inheritance in Man
  (OMIM), 59f, 59–60
Orkin, Stuart, 122–24, 124f
ornithine transcarbamylase (OTC) deficiency,
  107–8, 108f, 135–38
oversight
  emergence of, 85–90
  of recombinant DNA research, 91–97
  recommendations for, 185–88

p53 gene, 142
Pagano, Joseph, 85
pangenes, 24–27
pangenesis, intracellular, 24–27
papilloma virus, 61, 62–63
papovaviruses, 61, 64–65, 105, 106–7
Paracelsus, 9
Parvoviridae adeno-associated viruses, 112–13
Pasteur, Louis, 15, 17f, 17, 19, 189
Pasteur Institute, 67
patents, 121
pathology, cellular, 15
Pauling, Linus, 48–50, 53–54, 55f, 56f, 57
pentosuria, 31–34
peripheral artery disease, 143
Perutz, Max, 56–57
Pfizer, 99–101, 179–80
Pfizer-BioNTech, 179–80
Pfuderer, Peter, 61–62
pharma, 175–80
phenotype (term), 24–27, 37
Philippines, 143
PhiX174, 131
physician's handbook, 122f
plasmids, 143
*Points to Consider in the Design and Submission
  of Somatic Cell Human Gene Therapy
  Protocols*, 95, 119
polyethylene glycol (PEG), 120–21
polymerase chain reaction (PCR), 175–76

polyoma virus
  sequencing, 131
  vectors based on, 61, 63–65, 68–69, 105–7
Pompe's disease, 179–80
*Preclinical Data Development*, 95
President's Commission for the Study of Ethical Problems in Medicine and Biomedical and Behavioral Research, 95, 119–20
pricing, 181–82
prime editing, 166, 167, 173–74
prime-editing guide RNA (pegRNA), 167
Prime Medicine, 167
Princess of Asturia Prize, 179–80
*Proceedings of the Brünn Society for the Study of Natural Science*, 24
product replacement approach, 34–36, 141–42
programmable RNA-based RNA editing, 173–74
programmed cell death protein 1 gene (PDCD1), 163–64
provirus, 77–78
pseudoviruses, 63, 114–15
Ptolemy, 9
puerperal fever, 19–20

Qalsody (tofersen), 172–73
Qasim, Waseem, 159

randomized controlled trials (RCTs), 127, 129–30
Rawls, John, 183
Razes (Al-Razi), 9
recombinant DNA
  discovery of, 67–84
  first products to reach market, 176–77
  *NIH Guidelines for Research Involving Recombinant DNA Molecules*, 93–94, 95
  research oversight and regulation, 91–97, 92f
  SV-40-based gene transfer vector, 76–77
Recombinant DNA Advisory Committee (RAC), 93–95, 119
recombinant human growth hormone, synthetic, 176–77
recommendations, 185–88
Regeneron, 173
regulation
  emergence of, 85–90
  of recombinant DNA research, 91–97
  recommendations for, 185–88
Renaissance, 9–10
REPAIR (RNA editing for programmable adenosine replacement), 173–74
RESCUE (RNA editing for specific C-to-U exchange), 173–74

restriction enzymes, 70–77
retinal disease, 147–48, 172, 173
retroviruses
  foamy virus (FV), 115
  gammaretrovirus vectors, 119, 120, 146–47
  gene transfer tools, 108–12, 151
  terminology, 79
  reverse transcriptase, 70, 77–79, 81–84
Rexin-G, 143
Riggs, Arthur, 81–84, 176
RNA
  messenger RNA, 51, 67–68, 171–72
  prime-editing guide (pegRNA), 167
  programmable, 173–74
  role of, 51
  short hairpin RNAs (shRNAs), 171–72
  small interfering RNAs (siRNAs), 171–72, 173, 179–80
  transfer RNAs, 52
RNA-based therapies, 171–74
RNA editing
  programmable RNA-based, 173–74
  tools and targets, 171–73
RNA editing for programmable adenosine replacement (REPAIR), 173–74
RNA editing for specific C-to-U exchange (RESCUE), 173–74
Roblin, Richard, 69–70, 74f, 75f, 105–6
Roche, 179–80
Rockefeller Institute, 41–45
Rocktavian (BioMarin, Inc.), 179
Rogers, Stanfield, 61–63, 105
Rosenberg, Steven, 95, 96f, 119
Rous sarcoma virus, 77–78, 108–9
Royal Society (U.K.), 184–88
Royal Society of Science (England), 10–15
Royston, Ivor, 177
RPE65 gene, 147–48, 179
Russia, 143

Salk Institute, 63, 68–69, 105–6, 110–12, 131–32
Samulski, Richard Jude, 113, 116f
Sangamo Therapeutics, 158, 179–80
Sanger, Frederick (Fred), 56–57, 76–77, 79–81, 82f, 131, 189
Sanger dideoxy enzymatic sequencing technology, 79–81, 83f
San Raffaele Hospital (Milan, Italy), 146–47, 179–80
sarcoma
  bone, metastatic, 163–64
  CRISPR clinical trials for, 163–64
  Rous virus, 77–78, 108–9
Savulescu, Julian, 183

Schleiden, Matthias, 15
Schwann, Theodor, 15
Scolnick, Edward, 109*f*, 109–10
scurvy, 127
Second International Human Genome Editing Summit (2018), 183–84
Seemiller, Jay, 105–6
Semmelweiss, Ignaz, 15, 19–20, 20*f*, 189
sepsis, 19–20
severe combined immunodeficiency disease (SCID)
    ADA-SCID, 120–22, 146–47, 178
    gene therapy trials, 122–23, 129–30, 143–47, 144*f*, 178
    X-linked, 143
Sharpe, John Subak, 105–6
Sharpey-Schafer, Edward, 34
Shelley, Mary, 182–83
Shenzhen SiBiono GeneTech Co. Ltd., 142
Shope papilloma virus, 62–63
short hairpin RNAs (shRNAs), 171–72
sickle cell anemia, 53–57, 55*f*, 56*f*, 159
    CRISPR clinical trials, 164, 165
    treatment of, 165, 190
sickle cell disease
    CRISPR clinical trials, 164–65
    gene therapy for, 164–65
sickle cell hemoglobin (Hb-S), 54–57
sickle cell trait, 53–54, 55*f*
simian virus 40 (SV40)
    sequencing, 131
    vectors based on, 61, 63, 68–69, 76–77, 105–7
Singer, John, 53–54
Singer, Maxine, 91–92, 92*f*
Sinsheimer, Robert, 91, 105, 131–32
Skysona (elivaldogene autotemcel), 156
SMA (spinomuscular atrophy), 149–50, 172, 179
small interfering RNAs (siRNAs), 171–72, 173, 179–80
smallpox, 15–17
Smith, David, 131–32
Smith, Hamilton, 73–77, 75*f*, 189
Smithies, Oliver, 157
SMN1 (survival motor neuron) gene deficiency, 149–50
SMN1 (survival motor neuron) gene therapy, 172
somatostatin, 81–84, 176
Spark Therapeutics Inc., 179–80
speciation, de Vries concept of, 37–38
Spillman, William Jasper, 29*f*, 29
spinocerebellar ataxia type 3, 179–80

spinomuscular atrophy (SMA), 149–50, 172, 179
Spinraza (nusinersen), 149–50, 172
*Splicing Life*, 95
Spumaviruses, 108–9
St. Thomas Abbey (Brno), 24, 26*f*
Staehelin, Matthias, 57*f*
standards of care, 149–50
Stanford University, 67, 76–77
*Staphylococcus aureus*, 161–62
statins, 53
stem cells, hematopoietic (HPSCs), 164–65
sterilization, involuntary, 23–24
*Streptococcus pyogenes*, 161–62
*Streptococcus thermophilus*, 161–62
Strimvelis (MolMed), 147
superoxide dismutase (SOD1) gene, 172–73
surgery, aseptic, 19
survival motor neuron (SMN1) gene deficiency, 149–50
survival motor neuron (SMN1) gene therapy, 172
Sutton, Walter, 37
Sutton-Boveri chromosome theory, 37–40
SV40. *See* simian virus 40
Swanson, Robert, 176
"Swords into Plowshares" (Vuchetich), 64*f*
Syntex Corp., 99, 177
syphilis, 9, 128–29
Sysknus, Virginius, 161–62
Syskona, 181–82

T2 bacteriophage, 46
Takeda Pharmaceuticals, 179–80
TALENs (transcription activator-like effector nucleases), 159, 190
TALEs (transcription activator-like effectors), 158–59
TAL (transcription activator-like) nucleases, 157–58
Tatum, Edward, 42–43, 46*f*
T cell receptor transgenes, 163–64
technology
    biotechnology (biotech), 81–84, 164, 175–80
    recombinant DNA, 73–76
Telethon, 177–78, 179–80
Temin, Howard, 77–78, 78*f*, 108–10, 189
Terheggen, H.G., 62–63
Texas Children's Hospital, 143
thalassemia
    beta-thalassemia, 87–89, 158–59, 164–65, 181–82, 190

CRISPR clinical trials, 164-65
  gene therapy for, 164-65, 181-82, 190
  transfusion-dependent (TDT), 164-65
thalassophilia, 21-23
Theriac, 6-7
thin layer electrophoresis, 81f
thymidine kinase (TK), 85-87
T lymphocytes (T cells)
  chimeric antigen receptor (CAR), 150-52, 159, 189-90
  CRISPR-Cas9 PD-1-edited, 163
tobacco mosaic virus (TMV), 61-62
tofersen (Qalsody), 172-73
Tooze, John, 79
TP (transforming principle), 41
transcription, 67-68, 72f
transcription activator-like effector nucleases (TALENs), 159, 190
transcription activator-like effectors (TALEs), 158-59
transcription activator-like (TAL) nucleases, 157-58
transfection, 85-90
transfer RNAs, 52
transfusion-dependent thalassemia (TDT), 164-65
translation, 67-68, 72f
transposons, 39-40
"A Treatise on the Scurvy" (Lind), 127
Trono, Didier, 110-12, 113f
Tschermak, Erich von, 27f, 27-28
tuberculosis, 18, 129
tumor-infiltrating lymphocytes (TIL) cells, 119
tumor suppressor gene p53, 142
Tuskegee syphilis experiments, 128, 129
typhus, 18

UniQure, 156, 178-80
United States
  Department of Energy (DOE), 131-32
  federal oversight and regulation, 85-90
  Food and Drug Administration (FDA) (*see* Food and Drug Administration (FDA))
  Human Genome Project, 131-32
  National Academy of Sciences, 184-88
  National Commission for the Protection of Human Subjects of Biomedical and Behavioral Research, 129
  National Institutes of Health (NIH) (*see* National Institutes of Health (NIH))
University of Alicante, 160
University of California, Berkeley, 161-62, 184-85

University of California, Los Angeles (UCLA), 87-89, 139
University of California, San Diego (UCSD), 177
University of California, San Francisco, 77
University of California, Santa Cruz, 131-32
University of Florida, 113, 147-48
University of Heidelberg, 24
University of North Carolina, 157
University of Oxford, 183
University of Pennsylvania
  Gene Therapy Center, 135-39, 137f
  gene therapy trials, 99-101, 108f, 135-39, 147-48, 151-52
  Novartis alliance, 179-80
  pharma-biotech ventures, 179-80
University of Tübingen, 28
University of Umeå, 161-62
University of Utah, 157
University of Vienna, 161-62
University of Washington, 122-23
University of Wisconsin, 77-78, 109-10, 157
urinary tract infections, 166
Urnov, F., 158
U.S. Patent Office, 121
U.S. Public Health Service, 128
U.S. Supreme Court, 129
  *Buck v. Bell*, 23-24, 128, 182-83

vaccines
  development of, 179-80
  history of, 15-17
  mRNA-based, 99-101, 179-80
  Warp Speed program, 179-80
Vaheri, Antti, 85
Van der Eb, Alexander (Alex), 86, 87f
van Leeuwenhoek, Antonie, 10-15, 13f, 14f, 189
Varmus, Harold, 122-23, 129
vascular endothelial growth factor (VEGF), 143, 173
Venter, John Craig, 132f, 132-33
Verma, Inder, 110-12, 112f
Vertex, 164-65
Vesalius, Andreas, 10, 12f
vesicular stomatitis virus, 110-12
Vetter, David ("Texas bubble-boy"), 143, 144f
Vical Inc., 99, 101-3, 177, 179-80
Virchow, Rudolf, 15
Virginia
  *Buck v. Bell*, 23-24, 128, 182-83
  involuntary sterilization, 23-24

viruses
  bacterial (phages or bacteriophages), 43–46, 61, 76–77, 81*f*
  enteroviruses, recombinant, 115
  gene transfer vectors, 61–65, 70, 76–77, 105–6, 115
  nucleoside-modified mRNA-encoding antigens, 99–101
  papoviruses, 106–8
  provirus, 77–78
  pseudotyped or pseudoviruses, 63, 114–15
  retroviruses, 79, 108–12, 115, 119, 120, 146–47, 151
Vuchetich, Yeygeny, 64*f*

Waddington, Conrad, 38–39
Wagner, Ernst, 101, 102*f*
Warp Speed COVID vaccine program, 179–80
Watson, James, 49–50, 51*f*, 71*f*, 131–32, 189
WAVE, 173
WAVE Life Inc., 179–80
Weinberg, Robert, 109–10, 110*f*
Weissman, Drew, 99–101, 101*f*, 179–80
Weizmann Institute of Science (Israel), 151
Welch Medical Library (Johns Hopkins University), 59*f*, 59–60

Wells, Ibert, 53–54
Western concepts, early, 3–8
wet macular degeneration, 173
wild-type p53, 142
Wilkins, Maurice, 49–50, 50*f*
Willowbrook State Institution, New Jersey, 128, 129
Wilson, James, 135–37, 137*f*, 138–39
Wiskott-Aldrich Syndrome, 147
Wolff, Jon, 101–3, 103*f*
World War II, 128
WVE-004, 173

xenophobia, 21–23
*Xenopus*, 77
xeroderma pigmentosum, 159
X-linked SCID, 143
X-ray crystallography, 53–54

Zhang, Feng, 161–62
zinc (Zn)-finger base editing, 166–67, 190
zinc (Zn)-finger genome editing, 158–59
zinc (Zn)-finger nucleases, 157–59
Zinder, Norton, 91
Zolgensma (Novartis Gene Therapies, Inc.), 149–50, 172, 179
Zynteglo (LentiGlobin), 164–65, 181–82